Complementary Feeding: Building the Foundations for a Healthy Life

Nestlé Nutrition Institute Workshop Series

Vol. 87

Complementary Feeding: Building the Foundations for a Healthy Life

Editors

Robert E. Black Baltimore, MD, USA
Maria Makrides Adelaide, SA, Australia
Ken K. Ong Cambridge, UK

KARGER

Nestlé Nutrition Institute

Nestec Ltd., 55 Avenue Nestlé, CH–1800 Vevey (Switzerland)
S. Karger AG, P.O. Box, CH–4009 Basel (Switzerland) www.karger.com

Library of Congress Cataloging-in-Publication Data

Names: Nestlé Nutrition Workshop (87th : 2016 : Singapore), author. | Black, Robert E., editor. | Makrides, Maria, editor. | Ong, Ken, editor. | Nestlé Nutrition Institute, issuing body.
Title: Complementary feeding : building the foundations for a healthy life / editors, Robert E. Black, Maria Makrides, Ken K. Ong.
Description: Basel, Switzerland ; Karger ; Vevey, Switzerland : Nestle Nutrition Institute, [2017] | Series: Nestle Nutrition Institute workshop series, ISSN 1664-2147 ; vol. 87 | Includes bibliographical references and index.
Identifiers: LCCN 2016058415| ISBN 9783318059557 (hard cover : alk. paper) | ISBN 9783318059564 (e-ISBN)
Subjects: | MESH: Infant Nutritional Physiological Phenomena | Child Development | Congresses
Classification: LCC RJ216 | NLM WS 120 | DDC 649.33--dc23 LC record available at https://lccn.loc.gov/2016058415

Printed on acid-free and non-aging paper (ISO 9706)
ISBN 978–3–318–05955–7
e-ISBN 978–3–318–05956–4
ISSN 1664–2147
e-ISSN 1664–2155

KARGER Basel · Freiburg · Paris · London · New York · Chennai · New Delhi · Bangkok · Beijing · Shanghai · Tokyo · Kuala Lumpur · Singapore · Sydney

Contents

For more information on related publications, please consult the NNI website: www.nestlenutrition-institute.org

Preface

Good nutrition in the first 2 years of life is essential for the health and development of children with implications throughout life. Global recommendations are that babies be exclusively breastfed for 6 months and that breastfeeding be continued until at least 2 years, while complementary foods are to be introduced from about 6 months. Recognizing the importance of nutrition in young children, the 87th Nestle Nutrition Institute Workshop, which took place in Singapore on May 8–11, 2016, focused on complementary feeding as a foundation for healthy life. The objectives of the workshop were to share updates and recommendations on complementary feeding, as well as insights into strategies and interventions to promote healthy growth.

The first session of the workshop was an update on the evidence and practice of introducing complementary feeding, especially what foods and the timing of their use. *Merryn J. Netting* and *Maria Makrides* set the scene by highlighting the mismatch between complementary feeding guidelines and what often happens in practice across low- and middle-income countries as well as high-income countries. They outlined the key nutritional issues for infants during the complementary feeding period, especially the need for adequate iron and zinc. *Jacqueline F. Gould* continued the nutritional theme with her review of intervention studies of micronutrient supplementation or fortification during the complementary feeding period, and their effects on the developmental outcomes of children. Despite the importance of this topic, it was difficult to draw strong conclusions. Many of the available studies had extended intervention periods covering the period from pregnancy to mid-childhood, samples sizes were often small, and attrition was often high. *Jordan R. Green et al.* focused on the often forgotten area of textures of complementary foods and the need to match these to the oromotor development of the baby. They described sophisticated studies of chewing biomechanics to evaluate the age appropriateness of solid foods that vary in texture. The ultimate aim of these studies is to deliver science-based guidance regarding the safety and appropriateness of new foods, identifying children at risk for choking or feeding impairments, and designing new developmentally appropriate foods. Our focus then shifted to the role of when to introduce complementary foods, especially the more allergic foods, if we are to reduce the risk of childhood allergies. *Debra J. Palmer* provided a comprehensive update on the most recent evidence which suggests that all complementary foods, regardless of whether they are considered allergenic or not, can be introduced into infant diets from 6 months of age as the infant is developmentally ready. In the final presentation of the session, *Erin S. Ross* addressed taste and flavor development and highlighted that exposure to a wide variety of tastes during the complementary feeding period has a strong influence on the food repertoire later in childhood and may be an important foundation to a healthy and varied diet.

The second session was a consideration of the current situation in low- and middle-income countries where both weight and length gains are commonly less than expected based on World Health Organization global growth standards. This growth faltering may occur in the first 6 months of life, especially if exclusive breastfeeding is not practiced, but is most acute in the second 6 months of infancy when complementary foods are essential to provide a sufficient diet. This is also a period in which infants are exposed to many microbes and have frequent infectious diseases, which contribute to their growth deficits along with insufficient and poor-quality diets due to inadequate complementary feeding. Presentations in this session considered the current problems with complementary feeding, the general recommendations that need to be adapted to local practices and available foods, and the indicators that are being widely used for population level assessments of feeding practices. Evidence was considered on how much effect has been found with nutritional counseling interventions and with food supplements that are often targeted to food-insecure populations. The gains in growth demonstrated in community trials of these interventions justify their application, but also research to improve their implementation and to identify interventions that would provide larger effects. The importance of vitamins and minerals, collectively called micronutrients, has been recognized, and recent approaches have centered on their provision either in fortified commercial complementary foods or products that can be mixed into complementary foods at home. The latter include micronutrient powders and lipid-based micronutrient products. The current status of the evidence of their effects was reviewed. There is also substantial interest in ready-to-use complementary foods made with local food ingredients. The experience with such products that have been developed and used in Bangladesh and China were considered.

The third session discussed factors involved in complementary feeding that influence healthy growth and development in the context of an obesogenic environment. Hence, the emphasis was here on the prevention of rapid weight gain and the establishment of healthy eating habits. *Ken K. Ong* introduced the concept of early-life trajectories to later health. He described the wealth of evidence linking infancy weight gain to the risk of later obesity and discussed the underlying mechanisms. The recent advances in identifying genetic factors and infant appetite traits that contribute to these trajectories are leading to greater appreciation and understanding of parent-offspring interaction and signaling in infant feeding and weight gain. *Maureen M. Black* and *Kristen M. Hurley* analyzed the roles of the child and parent in infant feeding, and showed how the principles of responsive parenting can be applied to develop an approach to infant feeding that is responsive to infant cues but without the parent becoming indulgent to the child. They reported how interventions based on these principles may be applied to manage both infant food refusal and also infant overfeeding and obesity. *Lynne A. Daniels* described the development of such interventions in the context of anticipatory guidance to parents on the process of complementary feeding, which were tested in the NOURISH trial. While other large US trials are still in progress, she presented encouraging new data from the EPOCH study, a meta-analysis across four infant feeding trials in Australia and New Zealand. Finally, *Anne M. Dattilo* determined how infant feeding interventions might fit within a wider context of multicomponent early-life interventions that aim to change food- and diet-related behaviors, or feeding and associated lifestyle behaviors in the mother during pregnancy as well as in the infant and young child. Together, the session focused on early life as an important period for the development and prevention of obesity.

The format of the workshop was very conducive to discussion, and the participants were active in questioning the presenters and sharing their own experiences. As chairs of the workshop, and on behalf of all participants, we would like to thank Dr. *Natalia Wagemans* for the opportunity to highlight this subject of global importance. The arrangements were excellent and we also express our appreciation to the Nestlé Nutrition Institute and the local Nestlé team for the well-organized event.

Robert E. Black
Maria Makrides
Ken K. Ong

Foreword

The first 1,000 days of life, the time period from conception until 2 years of age, is the time in which the infant is the most vulnerable and which lays the foundation to its future health. The complementary feeding period from 6 to 24 months is part of the first 1,000 days during which infants undergo a huge developmental change with regard to bodily functions, personality, and will. The infant's energy needs and nutritional requirements will exceed that what breastfeeding can provide and the child is developmentally ready to receive solid foods. During this transitional period, infants also progress from exclusively milk-based liquid diet to the family diet and self-feeding. Thus, the complementary feeding period is not just an important time to satisfy an infant's nutrition, but also a time to form healthy food preferences and feeding practices, and to further stimulate the infant's future healthy development. Inappropriate complementary feeding can lead to inhibition of growth and development, to unhealthy food choices and eating habits, and/or result in childhood obesity, all of which have detrimental consequences for long-term health and survival of the child.

The 87th Nestlé Nutrition Institute Workshop, held from May 8–11, 2016, in Singapore, was entitled 'Complementary Feeding: Building the Foundations for a Healthy Life' and was a scientific platform for key stakeholders to discuss and engage in the latest cutting-edge research surrounding the transitional complementary feeding period.

The workshop program has been designed in a very comprehensive way to cover the complementary feeding period with all challenges and successful practices taking differences and variations in all parts of the world in consideration.

The first session led by Prof. *Maria Makrides* addressed a fundamental topic on the role of complementary feeding in healthy growth and development focusing on the timing and type of solid food introduction. While highlighting the differences between complementary feeding recommendation and the actual practices around the world it was shown that guidelines from different countries have many similar consistent and important themes, including complementary foods at/or around 6 months of age, continued breastfeeding, nutrient-dense complementary foods, hygienic food practices, development of feeding skills that nurture long-term healthy eating habits, and the prevention of micronutrient deficiencies and noncommunicable diseases such as obesity and allergy.

In the second session, chaired by Prof. *Robert E. Black*, the speakers examined the determinants of growth restriction and discussed effective interventions to improve complementary feeding practices and growth in infants and children in low- and middle-income countries. Determinants of these patterns of growth faltering include maternal factors (including age, height, and short birth intervals), pregnancy and birth conditions such as infections, and dietary factors. These factors contribute to fetal growth restriction, which put many infants on a lower growth trajectory. Dietary factors are important especially during the critical period of infancy as poor quality of complementary foods plays a vital role in growth faltering, while it can be prevented with dietary adequacy.

The last session led by Dr. *Ken K. Ong* has been focused on the importance and role of complementary feeding in development and 'programming' regarding behavioral and psychological aspects as well food preference in later life in high socioeconomic settings to prevent childhood obesity. The session discussion expanded on the topic of childhood obesity and modifiable risk factors associated with healthy growth as well as interventions addressing those associated with obesity prevention during the first 1,000 days. Childhood obesity is a strong predictor of adult obesity, and evidence from systematic reviews and meta-analyses suggests significant correlations between early childhood overweight, obesity, or measures of adiposity and modifiable factors during in utero development and early childhood. The importance of educating parents on the role of appropriate complementary feeding practices on long-term health outcome, building understanding and an open responsive environment during feeding time, helps parents to foster the child's developmental capacities and build a strong foundation for healthy life…

We would like to thank the three chairpersons *Maria Makrides, Robert E. Black* and *Ken K. Ong* for putting the scientific program together. We also would like to thank all speakers and scientific experts in the audience for their contributions to the content of the workshop as well as for scientific discussions. Finally, we thank Dr. *Grace Uy, Lin Angel, Christine Stillhart*, and their teams for their logistic support.

Dr. Natalia Wagemans
Head
Nestlé Nutrition Institute
Vevey, Switzerland

Contributors

Chairpersons & Speakers

Prof. Tahmeed Ahmed
Nutrition & Clinical Services
Services Division, icddr,b
68 Shahid Tajuddin Ahmed Sarani
Mahakhali, Dhaka 1212
Bangladesh
E-Mail tahmeed@icddrb.org

Prof. Marion Aw
College of Pediatrics & Child Health of Singapore
Division of Paediatric Gastroenterology Hepatology and Nutrition
National University Hospital
1E Kent Ridge Road
Singapore 119228
Singapore
E-Mail marion_aw@nuhs.edu.sg

Dr. Maureen M. Black
University of Maryland School of Medicine
737 W. Lombard Street, Room 161
Baltimore, MD 21201
USA
E-Mail mblack@peds.umaryland.edu

Prof. Robert E. Black
Institute for International Programs
Bloomberg School of Public Health
Johns Hopkins University
615 N Wolfe Street, Room E8545
Baltimore, MD 21205
USA
E-Mail rblack1@jhu.edu

Prof. Daisy Chan
Department of Neonatal and Developmental Medicine
Singapore General Hospital
Outram Road
Singapore 169608
Singapore
E-Mail daisy.chan.k.l@singhealth.com.sg

Prof. Lynne Allison Daniels
School of Exercise and Nutrition Sciences
Faculty of Health
Queensland University of Technology
Level 4, A Wing, O Block
Victoria Park Road
Kelvin Grove Campus, QLD 4059
Australia
E-Mail l2.daniels@qut.edu.au

Dr. Anne M. Dattilo
Nestlé Nutrition
Rue Entre-deux-Villes 10
CH–1800 Vevey
Switzerland
E-Mail anne.dattilo@us.nestle.com

Dr. Jacqueline F. Gould
Child Nutrition Research Centre
South Australian Health & Medical Research Institute (SAHMRI)
72 King William Road
Adelaide, SA 5000
Australia
E-Mail jacqueline.gould@adelaide.edu.au

Prof. Jordan R. Green
Communication Sciences and Disorders
MGH Institute of Health Professions
Charlestown Navy Yard
36 1st Avenue
Boston, MA 02129
USA
E-Mail jgreen2@mghihp.edu

Dr. Rebecca Heidkamp
Institute for International Programs &
Center for Human Nutrition
Bloomberg School of Public Health
Johns Hopkins University
615 N Wolfe Street, Room E2518
Baltimore, MD 21205
USA
E-Mail rheidka1@jhu.edu

Prof. Junsheng Huo
Department of Food Science and
Technology
Institute of Nutrition and Health, China
CDC
29 Nan Wei Road
Beijing 100050
China
E-Mail jshuo@263.net.cn

Prof. Yung Seng Lee
Department of Paediatrics
Yong Loo Lin School of Medicine
NUHS Tower Block, Level 12
1E Kent Ridge Road, Singapore 119228
Singapore
E-Mail yung_seng_lee@nuhs.edu.sg

Prof. Maria Makrides
Healthy Mothers, Babies and Children
South Australian Health & Medical
Research Institute (SAHMRI)
72 King William Road
Adelaide, SA 5000
Australia
E-Mail maria.makrides@sahmri.com

Dr. Lynnette M. Neufeld
Monitoring, Learning, Research
Global Alliance for Improved Nutrition
(GAIN)
Rue de Vermont 37–39
CH–1211 Geneva 20
Switzerland
E-Mail lneufeld@gainhealth.org

Dr. Ken K. Ong
MRC Epidemiology Unit
Institute of Metabolic Science
University of Cambridge
Cambridge Biomedical Campus
Box 285
Cambridge CB2 0QQ
UK
E-Mail ken.ong@mrc-epid.cam.ac.uk

Dr. Debra Jane Palmer
School of Paediatrics and Child Health
(SPACH)
University of Western Australia (M561)
35 Stirling Highway
Crawley, WA 6009
Australia
E-Mail debbie.palmer@uwa.edu.au

Prof. Victor Samuel Rajadurai
Department of Neonatology
KK Women's and Children's Hospital
100 Bukit Timah Road
Singapore 229899
Singapore
E-Mail victor.samuel@kkh.com.sg

Prof. Erin Sundseth Ross
Feeding FUNdamentals
12806 Forest Circle
Thornton, CO 80241
USA
E-Mail feedingfundamentals@gmail.
com

Dr. Marie T. Ruel
Poverty, Health and Nutrition Division
International Food Policy Research
Institute
2033 K Street, NW
Washington, DC 20006
USA
E-Mail m.ruel@cgiar.org

Participants

Merryn Netting/Australia
Karen Simmer/Australia
Greta Trent/Australia
Melinda White/Australia
Didarul Alam/Bangladesh
Mahbub Karim/Bangladesh
Mohammed Reaz Mobarak/Bangladesh

Milana Dan/Brazil
Eap Tekchheng/Cambodia
Zhang Lan/China
Zhenghong Li/China
Xiumei Liu/China
Hui Juan Ruan/China
Hannah Abou-El-Ghar/Egypt
Hisham Awad/Egypt
3Wael Bahbah/Egypt
Osama Elasheer/Egypt
Mohamed Nasreldin Elbarbary/Egypt
Wael Eltaei/Egypt
Mahmoud Elzalabany/Egypt
Emad Faltas/Egypt
Mohamed Ghazaly/Egypt
Moataza Hamed/Egypt
Tamer Hassan/Egypt
Adham Mohamed Eltahry Hegazy/Egypt
Hassan Heshmat/Egypt
Abdel Khalek Khalil/Egypt
Abdellatif Mohamed Abdelmoez Omar/Egypt
Vivian Tsang/Hong Kong
Devesh Agarwal/India
Gaurav Bhalla/India
Prasanta Kumar Datta/India
Satish Deopujari/India
Ashok Mohanlal Gawdi/India
Shamik Ghosh/India
Nomeeta Gupta/India
Mahesh Hiranandani/India
Jyotinder Kaur/India
Mahaboob Basha Kalluri/India
Dhananjay Kumar/India
Om Prakash Mahansaria/India
Prince Parakh/India
Savida Parameswaran/India
Shashidhar Rao/India
Srinivas Sankaranarayanan/India
Narmada Sheshadri/India
Ashish Kamaraj Shetty/India
Khaled Al-Sarraf/Kuwait
Kongkham Sisouk/Laos
Mona Alameh/Lebanon
Ziad El Hachem/Lebanon
Wai Seong Chin/Malaysia
Yao Mun Choo/Malaysia
George Keuh/Malaysia
Juan Loong Kok/Malaysia
Bee Swan Lee/Malaysia
Bee Koon Poh/Malaysia
Suhaida Abdul Rahman/Malaysia
Nor Azlina Mohammad Rashid/Malaysia
Rowani Mohd Rawi/Malaysia
Intan Nor Chahaya Shukor/Malaysia
Jimena De Martino/Mexico
Ameleen Bangayan/Philippines
Maria Gomez/Philippines
Almida Reodica/Philippines
Josephine Yuson-Sunga/Philippines
Mohammed Al-Hindi/Saudi Arabia
Abdelhai H. Hammo/Saudi Arabia
Musa Khormi/Saudi Arabia
Pauline Chan/Singapore
Mary Chong/Singapore
Mei Chien Chua/Singapore
Ciaran Forde/Singapore
Christiani Jeyakumar Henry/Singapore
Tingfei Ho/Singapore
Poh Choo Khoo/Singapore
Le Ye Lee/Singapore
Allan Lim/Singapore
Grace Lim/Singapore
Lilian Lim/Singapore
Steven Ng/Singapore
Ian Ong/Singapore
Lynette Shek/Singapore
Allyson Tan/Singapore
Nancy Tan/Singapore
Grace Uy/Singapore
Boh Boi Wong/Singapore
Fabian Yap/Singapore
She Shiang Yeoh/Singapore
Eurídice Castaneda Gutierrez/Switzerland
Sanjeev Ganguly/Switzerland
Yassaman Shahkhalili Dulloo/Switzerland
Simona Stan/Switzerland
Laurence Stoll-Le Guyader/Switzerland
Marco Turini/Switzerland
Nalinee Chongviriyaphan/Thailand
Umaporn Suthutvoravut/Thailand
Mohamed Khallaf/United Arab Emirates
Mohamed Sadik/United Arab Emirates
Rania Satouf/United Arab Emirates
Sarmad Farook Yahya/United Arab Emirates
Clare Llewellyn/UK
Pinki Sahota/UK
Anne Sidnell/UK
Randi Kline/USA
Tin Hoang Thi/Vietnam
Thuc Luu Thi My/Vietnam
Giang Nguyen Thi Linh/Vietnam

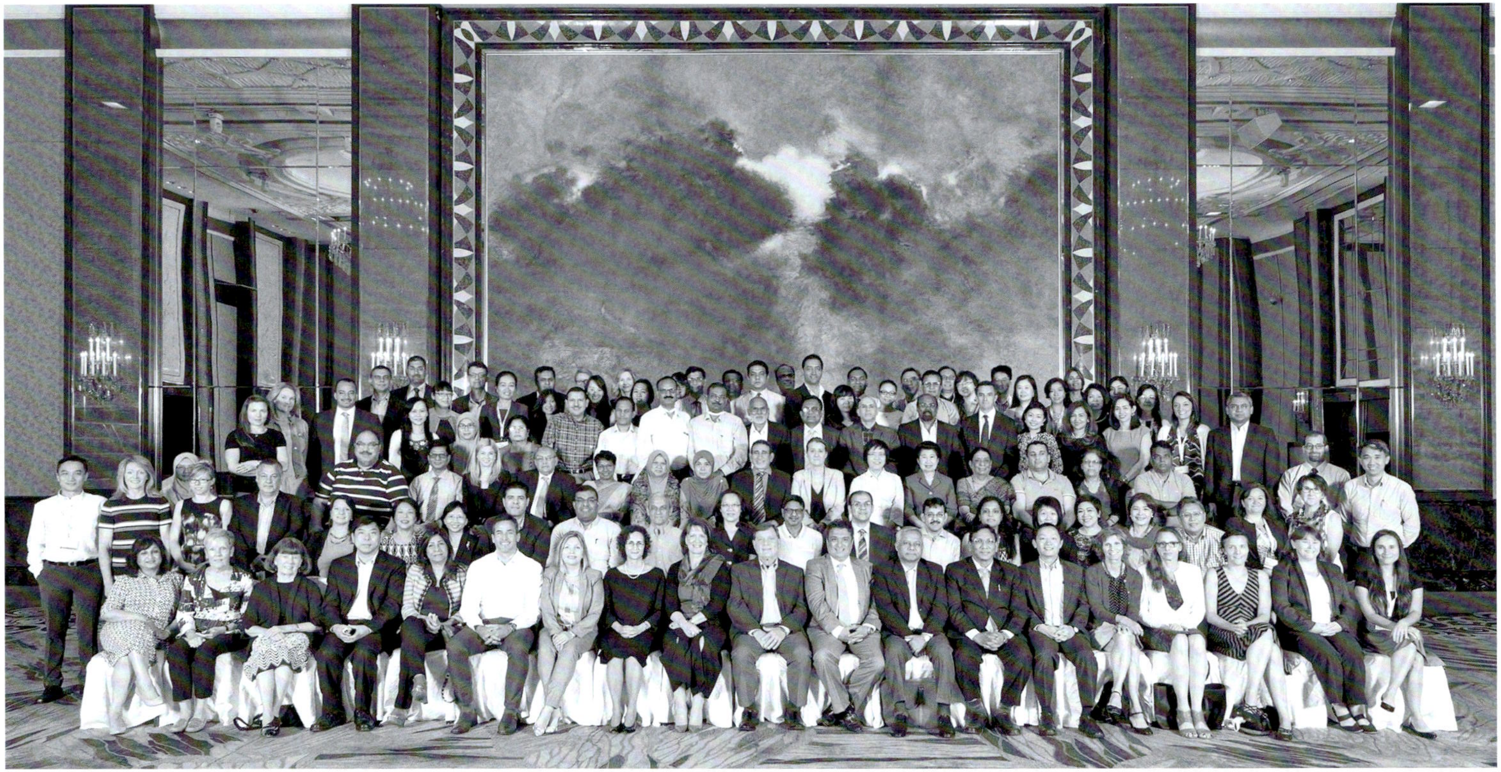

87th Nestlé Nutrition Institute Workshop
Singapore, May 8–11, 2016

Update on Introduction of Complementary Feeding

Black RE, Makrides M, Ong KK (eds): Complementary Feeding: Building the Foundations for a Healthy Life. Nestlé Nutr Inst Workshop Ser, vol 87, pp 1–12, (DOI: 10.1159/000449497)
Nestec Ltd., Vevey/S. Karger AG., Basel, © 2017

Complementary Foods: Guidelines and Practices

Merryn J. Netting[a, b] • Maria Makrides[a, b]

[a]Child Nutrition Research Centre, South Australian Health and Medical Research Institute (SAHMRI), and [b]Discipline of Pediatrics, School of Medicine, The University of Adelaide, Adelaide, SA, Australia

Abstract

Complementary feeding, the transition from a breast milk-based diet to inclusion of other sources of nutrition in an infant's diet, is a major milestone in infant development. This transition period is important as it is a time when infants are vulnerable to developing nutritional deficiencies and occurs during a developmental stage when important food-related behavioral patterns are being established. As under- and overnutrition may coexist in children from the same country, it is important that advice provided by complementary feeding guidelines meets the needs of all children helping them to grow and develop into healthy adults. Many consistent and important themes emerge when comparing complementary feeding guidelines from different countries: complementary foods at or around 6 months of age; continued breastfeeding; nutrient-dense complementary foods; hygienic food practices; development of feeding skills that foster long-term healthy eating habits, and prevention of non-communicable diseases such as obesity. Complementary feeding guidelines that promote good eating during the first year and beyond recognize that nutrition, particularly during the first 1,000 days, has an important influence on immediate growth and development, but also an important role in setting up taste preferences and behavioral patterns which inform an infant's susceptibility to development of disease later in life. However, guidelines in many countries are not always followed, particularly during the second year of life, and innovative methods are needed to increase compliance.

Introduction

Complementary feeding, the transition from a breast milk-based diet to inclusion of other sources of nutrition in an infant's diet, is a major milestone in infant development. This transition period occurs at a time when infants are vulnerable to developing nutritional deficiencies during a developmental stage when long-term behavioral patterns are being established. The complementary feeding period extends from the early initiation phase to establishing meal and food habits that will move with the infant into early childhood and beyond.

In low- and middle-income countries, the focus of complementary feeding recommendations is to prevent growth faltering caused by delayed complementary feeding or inadequate feeding practices, where too little food is offered or the food is of low nutrient density. This is in contrast to high income countries where malnutrition caused by improper feeding behavior and poor food choices may present as under- or overnutrition. There is an increasing body of evidence that early feeding, particularly during the first 1,000 days, plays an important influence in setting up food preferences and eating behaviors that will influence a child's susceptibility to non-communicable diseases later in life. As such, it is important to provide guidelines that prevent chronic disease influenced by early nutrition.

We aim to compare official feeding recommendations as they apply in low-, middle- and high-income countries, and to discuss current evidence related to feeding practices as obtained from dietary intake surveys. The consequences of feeding complementary foods too early or too late will be discussed, and knowledge gaps and opportunities for further research identified.

Infant/Toddler/Child: Changing Requirements for Growth and Development

Breastfeeding is the gold standard for infant feeding, and it is encouraged for 2 years and beyond, as long as the mother and child desire [1]. However, at around 6 months of age, an infant's requirements for energy, protein and other nutrients (particularly iron and zinc) cannot be met by breast milk alone [1]. At around the same time, infants begin to demonstrate signs that they are developmentally ready to begin eating solid foods as the tongue thrust reflex is lost and they start to show interest in the food that people around them are eating. Infants may watch when others are eating, opening their mouths for food, or they may reach for food on a parent's or caregiver's plate. Parents may naturally respond to these signs by offering the child a small amount of the food from their plate or by consciously making the decision to start to offer their child complementary foods. Foods offered may be home prepared or commercially available infant foods. Foods may be placed into the infant's mouth using clean fingers, offered from a spoon, or the baby may be encouraged to feed itself. Regardless of which foods are given and the manner in which they are offered, the early feeding environment begins to establish longer-term attitudes and eating behaviors.

The appropriate timing of introduction to complementary foods is often called the 'window of opportunity'. This window may be considered in terms of specific nutritional requirements at the time, as a developmental opportunity in terms of receptiveness to varied textures of foods [2], or may be considered as optimal timing of exposure to food allergens to foster development of immune tolerance [3].

Around a child's first birthday, there is a relative (per kilo) drop in energy and protein requirements associated with decreased growth velocity. However, requirements for many micronutrients (specifically, vitamins B_1, B_2, B_3, B_6, B_{12} and calcium) increase from the first to the second year, while needs for others (in particular iron, zinc and iodine) remain similar to those at 6–12 months [4, 5]. During this stage, the nutritional quality of the food in the child's diet becomes even more important as relatively less food is required to maintain growth, for example per 100 calories of food, a 6- to 8-month-old breastfed infant's iron requirement is estimated to be equivalent to 9 times that of an adult male [5].

In addition to meeting specific nutritional requirements, this time comes at a delicate developmental stage as the child begins to focus on development of gross motor skills and begins to assert independence. During the toddler period at 12–24 months of age, mealtimes may become difficult, and food neophobia may become an issue with many toddlers preferring familiar foods presented in the same way [6]. This, coupled with potential parental concern related to slow growth and perceived picky eating, can lead to a 'perfect storm' of control related to mealtimes and eating. When managing potential feeding issues, a balance between too-controlling and laissez-faire parenting leads to the best behavioral outcomes [7]. Parents can help young children develop good eating patterns by establishing a meal and snack time routine, offering a variety of foods as part of a healthy diet and allowing the child to control which foods from the meal or snack they eat in amounts that satisfy their appetite [8].

Eventually the toddler becomes a preschooler and then a school-age child. Optimal nutrition remains important during each of these stages as early eating habits often translate into lifelong eating patterns and eventually influence long-term health outcomes.

How Do We Meet These Changing Needs as Children Grow and Develop? Complementary Feeding Guidelines and Policies

Infant feeding guidelines, including instructions related to complementary feeding, are developed by many countries and are underpinned by the global nutrition strategies of the World Health Organization (WHO), which primarily aim to prevent undernutrition in low- and middle-income countries. The WHO advocates for exclusive breastfeeding for 6 months and complementary feeding from 6 months of age, with continued breastfeeding until 2 years of age. This advice has recently been strengthened by the WHO, restating that these guidelines are applicable for both low-/middle-income as well as high-income countries [1, 9].

Despite traditional feeding practices and health issues specific to each country or region, there are many common themes in these feeding guidelines (summarized in table 1).

Exclusive Breastfeeding

Breastfeeding is recommended in all feeding guidelines surveyed; however, recommendations surrounding length of exclusive breastfeeding vary in subtle ways, related to the recommended timing of introduction to complementary foods.

Timing of Complementary Foods

The wording used to describe the timing of introduction to complementary foods is at, from or after 6 months [1, 10–18] or, approximately, around 6 months of age [19–21]. Where complementary feeding prior to 6 months of age is included in the guidelines there is general agreement that complementary feeding should not commence prior to 4 months of age due to the increased risk of obesity, gastrointestinal disorders and development of allergy [19, 20]. Most countries include the importance of waiting for developmental cues pertaining to 'readiness' for complementary foods, and some include guidelines related to responsive feeding, where the infants feeding cues are observed and followed by the parent or caregiver. Developmental cues rather than a specific age may be the best indicator of 'readiness' to accept complementary foods.

Continued Breastfeeding with Complementary Foods

Breastfeeding is encouraged during the complementary feeding period because of its nutrient profile, beneficial effect on the gut microbiome, protection from infection, and longer-term benefits to maternal health [22].

Types of Complementary Foods

The recommended types of first complementary foods vary slightly from country to country, but nutrient-dense, iron-rich foods are universally encouraged as iron deficiency disorders are a major health issue in both low-/middle- and high-income countries. In many countries, iron-fortified cereals are recommended,

Table 1. Themes used for complementary feeding guidelines by organisation and country

Theme	Country or organisation
Exclusive breastfeeding	
For the first 6 months of life	WHO/UNICEF [1]; USA (AAP) [10]: Canada [11]; Brazil [12]; Sub-Saharan Africa [13]; India [14]; Philippines [15]; Hong Kong [16]; Singapore [17]; Malaysia [18]
For about/around 6 months	ESPGHAN [19]; Australia [20]; NZ [21]
Continued breastfeeding	
At least 1 year or beyond	NZ [21]
Until 2 years or beyond	WHO/UNICEF [1]; Australia [20]; Canada [11]; Brazil [12]; Sub-Saharan Africa [13]; India [14]; Malaysia [18]
Complementary foods	
Timing	
At/from/after 6 months	WHO/UNICEF [1]; USA (NIH) [29]; Canada [11]; Sub-Saharan Africa [13]; India [14]; Philippines [15]; Singapore (181 days) [17]; Malaysia [18]
At approximately/around 6 months	USA (AAP) [10]; Australia [20]; NZ [21]; Hong Kong [16]
Not before 17 or after 26 weeks	ESPGHAN [19]
When 'developmentally ready'	NZ [21]
Types	
Meet energy/protein needs	USA (AAP) [10]; Philippines [15]
Foods high in iron	USA: AAP [10] and NIH (cereal) [29]; Australia [20]; NZ (+ vitamin C) [21]; Canada [11]; Singapore [17]; Malaysia [18]
Foods high in zinc	USA (AAP) [10]
Nutrient-dense foods	Sub-Saharan Africa (vitamin A, zinc, iron, iodine) [13]; Philippines (micronutrients) [15]
Consistency increasing with age	WHO/UNICEF [1]; Australia [20]; NZ [21]; Canada [11]; Brazil [12]; Malaysia [18]
A variety of foods	WHO/UNICEF [1]; USA (AAP)[a] [10]; Australia [20]; NZ [21]; Canada [11]; Brazil [12]
Specify how often and how much	WHO/UNICEF [1][b]; USA (NIH) [29]; NZ [21]; Canada [11]; Brazil [12]; Sub-Saharan Africa [13]; Malaysia [18]
Specific food ideas	USA (NIH) [29]; Brazil [12]; Hong Kong (foods from family food basket) [16]; Singapore [17]; Malaysia [18]
Use fortified complementary foods	WHO/UNICEF [1]; Australia (iron) [20]; Canada [11]
Vitamin/mineral supplements as needed	WHO/UNICEF [1]; Sub-Saharan Africa [13]; India [14]; Philippines (vitamin A, iron, iodine) [15]
Other themes	
Responsive feeding	WHO/UNICEF [1]; USA (AAP) [10]; USA (NIH) [29]; Canada [11]; Brazil [12]; Hong Kong [16]; Malaysia [18]
Self-feeding	USA (AAP) [10]; Canada [11]; Malaysia [18]
Progression to healthy family foods	Australia [20]; NZ [21]; Brazil [12]
Hygienic food preparation and handling	WHO/UNICEF [1]; USA (AAP [10]; NIH [29]); Australia [20]; Canada [11]; Brazil [12]; Sub-Saharan Africa [13]; India [14]
Guidelines for feeding during illness	WHO/UNICEF [1]; Brazil [12]; India [14]; Malaysia [18]
No added salt, sugar, nutrient-poor foods	USA (NIH) [29]; Australia [20]; NZ [21]; Brazil [12]; Malaysia [18]

Table 1. Continued

Theme	Country or organisation
Limited or no juice	USA (AAP) [10]; NZ [21]; Malaysia [18]
Choking risk foods	USA (NIH) [29]; Australia [20]; Canada [11]
Monitor growth	USA (AAP) [10]
Physical activity	NZ [21]
Malnutrition/nutrient deficiencies	Sub-Saharan Africa [13]; India [14]; Philippines [15]
Allergy prevention	
Too early increases risk	Hong Kong [16]
Do not delay allergens	USA (AAP) [10]; ESPGHAN; Australia [20]
Delay/avoid allergens	USA (NIH) [29]; Malaysia (egg white after 1 year of age) [18]; Singapore [17]

AAP = American Academy of Pediatrics. New Zealand (NZ) guidelines include toddlers. Philippines – locally produced, low-cost foods.

[a] Foods from each food group by 7 months [USA (AAP)].

[b] 2–3 meals per day for infants 6–8 months of age and 3-4 meals per day for infants 9–23 months of age, with 1–2 additional snacks as required (WHO). NZ guidelines include toddlers. Philippines – locally produced, low-cost foods.

although many countries now encourage early inclusion of other iron-rich foods, including meat [23], egg [24] and legumes, in the infant's diet.

Delaying cord clamping after birth, a non-nutritional strategy has also been identified for reducing the incidence of iron deficiency. Delayed cord clamping for more than a minute after birth, or until the cord stops pulsing, is recommended by the WHO [25] as a strategy for increasing early hemoglobin concentrations and iron stores in infants [26].

Hygienic Food Practices

Food-borne illness is an important public health issue worldwide [27]. Recommendations related to safe food hygiene considerations are included in many infant feeding guidelines, and include instructions on hand washing, safe food preparation and food storage.

Development of Long-Term Feeding Skills

Progression from thick spoon foods to mashed foods and finger foods, and consumption of nutritious family foods are highlighted in many of the complementary feeding guidelines surveyed. Thick spoon foods are recommended for their energy and nutrient density, as compared with thin gruels. Exposure to thicker and lumpier foods is also important as this enables an infant to develop the oromotor skills that will enable them to eat the range of food textures required to transition to family meals [28]. Many infant feeding guidelines encourage caregivers to follow the child's feeding cues to foster independent eating skills and development of good mealtime habits.

Learning to Eat a Healthy Diet

Non-communicable diseases, including obesity and diabetes, are increasingly prevalent in both low-/middle- and high-income countries. Accordingly, early feeding guidelines from several countries are now attempting to address these issues, e.g. specific guidelines to not add sugar, salt or extra fat to complementary foods. Limiting or avoiding energy-dense drinks such as juice is also noted in many infant feeding guidelines [12, 18, 20, 21, 29].

These recommendations are accompanied by guidelines related to responsive feeding aiming to prevent parents from overfeeding their infants and teaching children positive mealtime behaviors that will set up longer-term eating patterns. The New Zealand Ministry of Health has taken this as an extra step, including also specific guidelines for physical activity, in their infant and toddler feeding guidelines [21].

Guidelines to Prevent Immune-Specific Outcomes

There is a progression from guidelines related to meeting basic nutritional needs to the development of guidelines related to non-nutritional outcomes. Guidelines targeting early feeding to prevent immune-based diseases (allergy and coeliac disease) have been released by Australian, European and American expert bodies [30–32]. Recent infant feeding guidelines for the prevention of allergy recommend exclusive breastfeeding until complementary feeding commences, and actively promote earlier introduction of common allergens (specifically peanut) into the infant's diet (from 4 months onwards as opposed to delayed introduction) [30, 31]. The European Society for Paediatric Gastroenterology, Hepatology and Nutrition (ESPGHAN) and North American Society for Pediatric Gastroenterology, Hepatology and Nutrition guidelines for infants genetically at risk of developing coeliac disease state that gluten may be introduced into the infant's diet anytime between 4 and 12 completed months of age and that consumption of large quantities of gluten should be avoided during the first weeks after gluten introduction and during infancy [32].

Are the Guidelines Being Followed? What Is Happening at Home?

Feeding guidelines are interpreted by the infant's caregiver in the context of their cultural, societal and economic circumstances and translated into the actual food offered, and how it is fed to the child. Surveys assessing effectiveness of national feeding guidelines are performed regularly in many countries, and, when performed sequentially, the results of these surveys may be used to describe changes over time. Many surveys collect information related to breastfeeding commencement rates and duration of exclusive breastfeeding. Some feeding surveys collect information related to the timing of complementary foods; however, the type and amounts of complementary foods consumed are not always described.

In low-/middle-income countries, early complementary feeding (prior to 4 months of age) and delayed complementary feeding (after 6 months of age) have been identified as issues of concern. In India, less than half (44%) of the infants from rural and urban slums commence complementary feeding at 6–8 months of age [33], whereas initiation of complementary feeding at 6 months of age was reported by 78% urban families of higher socioeconomic status and levels of education [33]. Likewise, in the Philippines, just over half (58%) of 6- 10-month-old infants are given timely, adequate and safe complementary foods [34]. On the other hand, data from 14 of 19 countries in Latin America and the Caribbean suggest that less than half of infants are exclusively breastfed at 6 months of age indicating that they had already commenced complementary feeding or were on other forms of milk [35]. The timing of complementary feeding and the types of food offered are related to cultural feeding practices, socioeconomic status and education levels of the parents [33]. Feeding surveys should collect information related to both the timing of complementary feeding and the types of foods consumed as there is some indication that as countries become more industrialized infants are offered foods of high fat and sugar content along with sugary drinks.

In higher-income countries, while complementary feeding prior to 4 months of age is common in some countries [36], most children commence complementary feeding from 4 to around 6 months of age, consistent with recommendations for timing of complementary feeding around 6 months of age. In the USA, information from the 2008 Feeding Infants and Toddlers Study (FITS 2008) indicates that although exclusive breastfeeding at 6 months of age is rare, infants are being breastfed longer (49% at 6 months and 24% at 12 months) [37]. The 2010 Australian National Infant Feeding survey (a longitudinal survey of 52,000 infants) reported 60.1% of infants surveyed were receiving breast milk at 6 months of age, with 34.6% of 4-month-old and only 3.9% of 6-month-old infants exclusively breastfed having started complementary feeding during this period. At 3 months 9.7%, at 4 months 35.3% and at 6 months 91.5% had consumed soft, semi-solid or solid foods in the 24 h before the survey [38].

When the type of foods consumed by infants is considered, feeding studies from the USA and Australia indicate that most of the infants and toddlers consume nutritionally adequate diets, but a small number of older infants are not getting enough iron and zinc indicating the feeding transition from late infancy to 2 years of age is an issue. Low intake of fruits and vegetables and frequent consumption of 'discretionary foods' high in fat, sugar and salt have been identified. In the American cohort described in FITS 2008, intake of fruits and vegetables was low, with 10.9% of 1-year-olds and 8.7% of 2-year-olds consuming dark green vegetables, 24.4% of 1-year-olds and 15.4% of 2-year-olds consuming deep yellow vegetables [39]. Fried potato products, including French fries, were consumed by 18.5% of 1-year-olds and 16.7% of 2-year-olds on a daily basis. Discretionary foods with high sugar and fat content were also consumed regularly by many of the young children surveyed with 40% of 1- and 2-year-olds consuming cakes, pies, cookies and pastries at least once a day; 6.6% of 1-year-olds and 31.8% of 2-year-olds consuming candy at least once per day, and 10.4% of 1-year-olds and 23.7% of 2-year-olds consuming salty snacks (including potato crisps and corn chips) at least once a day [39]. Similarly, in Australia a cross-sectional survey of 1- to 5-year-old pre-school children in Adelaide reported that even though children achieved the estimated average requirement for key micronutrients, including iron, zinc, calcium and vitamin C, they also consumed excessive amounts of saturated fat from biscuits, sweet buns, cakes, pastry and processed meat [40].

Although infants in middle- and upper-income countries are initially fed well, a mismatch begins to develop between the feeding guidelines and foods consumed by young children during their second and third years of life. Reasons for this discrepancy are not well documented, but may include underlying parental anxiety related to their child's growth, concern that the child is not eating enough, and the desire to see a child eat regardless of the nutritional quality of the food [6]. The child on the other hand may simply want to eat the same foods as other members of the household, and the results of feeding surveys may simply reflect household diets. Consumption of energy-dense high-fat, high-sugar 'discretionary foods' from an early age contribute to the risk of obesity and sets the trajectory of taste preferences and behavior that may contribute to the later onset of non-communicable diseases [41]. Given the natural progression of infant to toddler to child, complementary feeding guidelines directed at infants and toddlers should facilitate the development of skills underpinning the dietary guidelines for children, such as learning to eat a variety of healthy foods.

Summary and Conclusion

Early life nutrition, particularly during the first 1,000 days, has an important influence on immediate growth and development, but also an important role in forming early food preferences and food behavior that set the trajectory to susceptibility to development of non-communicable disease later in life.

In low-/middle income countries, existing complementary feeding guidelines emphasize avoidance of undernutrition specifically focusing on continued breastfeeding, and commencement of nutritious foods at the right time. In higher-income countries although infants are initially given nutrient-rich foods, there soon becomes a mismatch between the guidelines and feeding practices as discretionary foods high in fat, salt and sugar begin to appear early in the child's diet often before the second year of life [39, 40]. This pattern is also beginning to be seen in some low-/middle-income countries as more commercial foods become available [35]. This is of concern as eating patterns and food preferences established early in life are carried into adulthood [42], and early obesity leads to greater risk of non-communicable disease later in life.

It is not known if these eating patterns develop simply because they reflect the foods that are consumed by the rest of the household, or if caregivers offer these foods to young children due to perceived dislike of plain foods low in sugar or fat. Complementary feeding guidelines that encouraging positive feeding behaviors will help support caregivers to teach infants and young children to eat well.

Activity guidelines, including recommendations related to 'screen time' are beginning to appear as part of early feeding guidelines, and are important as these reflect the importance of both healthy eating and an active lifestyle. Early feeding guidelines should begin to reflect healthy eating and activity guidelines seen in guidelines for children, adolescents and adults as the early feeding period is important for setting early taste preferences and informing long-term behavioral patterns. However, innovative methods and significant advances in implementation science will be needed to maximize adoption of the guidelines.

Disclosure Statement

M.M. is an NHMRC (National Health and Medical Research Council) Principal Research Fellow and serves on scientific advisory boards for Nestlé and Fonterra. Associated honoraria are paid to her institution to support conference travel and continuing education for postgraduate students and early career researchers. No other disclosures were reported.

References

1 WHO/UNICEF: Global Strategy for Infant and Young Child Feeding. Geneva, World Health Organization, 2003.

2 Northstone K, Emmet P, Nethersole F, et al: The effect of age of introduction to lumpy solids on foods eaten and reported feeding difficulties at 6 and 15 months. J Hum Nutr Diet 2011;14:43–54.

3 Prescott SL, Smith P, Tang M, et al: The importance of early complementary feeding in the development of oral tolerance: concerns and controversies. Pediatr Allergy Immunol 2008;19:375–380.
4 Dewey KG: The challenge of meeting nutrient needs of infants and young children during the period of complementary feeding: an evolutionary perspective. J Nutr 2013;143: 2050–2054.
5 Dewey KG, Brown KH: Update on technical issues concerning complementary feeding of young children in developing countries and implications for intervention programs. Food Nutr Bull 2003;24:5–28.
6 Dovey TM, Staples PA, Gibson EL, Halford JC: Food neophobia and 'picky/fussy' eating in children: a review. Appetite 2008;50:181–193.
7 Manikam R, Perman JA: Pediatric feeding disorders. J Clin Gastroenterol 2000;30:34–46.
8 Satter E: How to get your kid to eat.... but not too much. Palo Alto, Bull Publishing, 1987.
9 Perkin MR, Logan K, Tseng A, et al: Randomized trial of introduction of allergenic foods in breast-fed infants. N Engl J Med 2016;374:1733–1743.
10 American Academy of Pediatrics Committee on Nutrition: Pediatric Nutrition, ed 7. Elk Grove Village, American Academy of Pediatrics, 2014.
11 Health Canada, Canadian Pediatric Society, Dietitians of Canada, & Breastfeeding Committee for Canada. Nutrition for healthy term infants: Recommendations from six to 24 months. http://www.hc-sc.gc.ca/fn-an/nutrition/infant-nourisson/recom/recom-6–24-months-6–24-mois-eng.php#a12014 (accessed May 2, 2016).
12 Brazil/Ministerio de Saúde: Guia alimentar para crianças menores de 2 anos. Serie A. Normas e manuais técnicos no 107. J Pediatr (Rio J) 2004;80:S131–S141.
13 Wuehler SE, Hess SY, Brown KH: Accelerating improvements in nutritional and health status of young children in the Sahel region of Sub-Saharan Africa: review of international guidelines on infant and young child feeding and nutrition. Matern Child Nutr 2011; 7(suppl 1):6–34.
14 Infant and Young Child Feeding Chapter, Indian Academy of Pediatrics, Rajeshwari K, et al: Infant and young child feeding guidelines: 2010. Indian Paediatr 2010;47:995–1004.
15 Department of Health, Republic of the Philippines: Administrative Order 2005-0014 National Policies of Infant and Young Child Feeding, 2005.
16 Department of Health, The Government of the Hong Kong Special Administrative Region: Report on Infant Feeding. 2014. http://www.fhs.gov.hk/english/reports/index.html (accessed March 21, 2016).
17 Singapore Government Health Promotion Board. Baby's First Food Journey http://www.hpb.gov.sg/HOPPortal/article?id=2728 (accessed March 21, 2016).
18 National Coordinating Committee on Food and Nutrition, Ministry of Health Malaysia: Malaysia Dietary Guidelines for Children and Adolescents. 2013.
19 Agostoni C, Decsi T, Fewtrell M, et al: Complementary feeding: a commentary by the ESPGHAN Committee on Nutrition. J Pediatr Gastroenterol Nutr 2008;46:99–110.
20 National Health and Medical Research Council, Australia: Infant Feeding Guidelines: Summary. Canberra, National Health and Medical Research Council, 2013.
21 New Zealand Ministry of Health: Food and Nutrition Guidelines for Healthy Infants and Toddlers (Aged 0–2): A Background Paper, partially revised December 2012. Wellington, Ministry of Health, 2008.
22 Victoria CG, Bahle R, Barros AJD, et al: Breastfeeding in the 21st century: epidemiology, mechanisms, and lifelong effect. Lancet 2016;387:475–490.
23 Krebs NF, Wescott JE, Butler N, et al: Meat as a first complementary food for breastfed infants: feasibility and impact on zinc intake and status. J Pediatr Gastroenterol Nutr 2006; 42:207–214.
24 Makrides M, Hawkes JS, Neumann MA, Gibson RA: Nutritional effect of including egg yolk in the weaning diet of breast-fed and formula-fed infants: a randomized controlled trial. Am J Clin Nutr 2002;75:1084–1092.
25 WHO: Guideline: Delayed Umbilical Cord Clamping for Improved Maternal and Infant Health and Nutrition Outcomes. Geneva, WHO, 2014.

26 McDonald SJ, Middleton P, Dowswell T, Morris PS: Effect of timing of umbilical cord clamping of term infants on maternal and neonatal outcomes. Cochrane Database Syst Rev 2013;7:CD004074.
27 WHO: WHO Estimates of the Global Burden of Foodborne Diseases: Foodborne Diseases Burden Epidemiology Reference Group 2007-201. Geneva, WHO, 2015.
28 Green RJ, Samy G, Miqdady MS, et al: How to improve eating behaviour during early childhood. Pediatr Gastroenterol Hepatol Nutr 2015;18:1–9.
29 United States of America National Institute of Health: Feeding Patterns and Diet – Children 6 Months to 2 Years. 2015. https://www.nlm.nih.gov/medlineplus/ency/patientinstructions/000713.htm (accessed May 2, 2016).
30 Fleischer DM, Sicherer S, Greenhawt M, et al: Consensus communication on early peanut introduction and the prevention of peanut allergy in high-risk infants. World Allergy Organ J 2015;8:27.
31 Australasian Society for Clinical Immunology and Allergy: ASCIA Infant Feeding Advice 2016. http://www.allergy.org.au/health-professionals/papers/ascia-infant-feeding-advice (accessed May 3, 2016).
32 Szajewska H, Shamir R, Mearin L, et al: Gluten Introduction and the Risk of Coeliac Disease: A Position Paper by the European Society for Pediatric Gastroenterology, Hepatology, and Nutrition. J Pediatr Gastroenterol Nutr 2016;62:507–513.
33 Kuriyan R, Kurpad AV: Complementary feeding patterns in India. Nutr Metab Cardiovasc Dis 2012;22:799–805.
34 Department of Health, Republic of the Philippines: Philippine IYCF Strategic Plan of Action for 2011–2016. 2011.
35 Lutter CK: Growth and complementary feeding in the Americas. Nutr Metab Cardiovasc Dis 2012;22:806–812.
36 Caroli M, Mele RM, Tomaselli MA, et al: Complementary feeding patterns in Europe with a special focus on Italy. Nutr Metab Cardiovasc Dis 2012;22:813–818.
37 Dwyer JT, Butte NF, Deming DM, et al: Feeding Infants and Toddlers Study 2008: progress, continuing concerns, and implications. J Am Diet Assoc 2010;110:S60–S67.
38 Australian Institute of Health and Welfare: 2010 Australian National Infant Feeding Survey: Indicator Results. Canberra, Australian Institute of Health and Welfare, 2011.
39 Siega-Riz AM, Deming DM, Reidy KC, et al: Food consumption patterns of infants and toddlers: where are we now? J Am Diet Assoc 2010;110:S38–S51.
40 Zhou SJ, Gibson RA, Gibson RS, Makrides M: Nutrient intakes and status of preschool children in Adelaide, South Australia. Med J Aust 2012;196:696–700.
41 Adair LS: How could complementary feeding patterns affect the susceptibility to NCD later in life? Nutr Metab Cardiovasc Dis 2012;22:765–769.
42 Mikkila V, Rasanen L, Raitakari OT, et al: Consistent dietary patterns identified from childhood to adulthood: the cardiovascular risk in Young Finns Study. Br J Nutr 2005;93:923–931.

Black RE, Makrides M, Ong KK (eds): Complementary Feeding: Building the Foundations for a Healthy Life. Nestlé Nutr Inst Workshop Ser, vol 87, pp 13–28, (DOI: 10.1159/000448934)
Nestec Ltd., Vevey/S. Karger AG., Basel, © 2017

Complementary Feeding, Micronutrients and Developmental Outcomes of Children

Jacqueline F. Gould

South Australian Health and Medical Research Institute, Adelaide, SA, Australia

Abstract

The period of complementary feeding (6–24 months of age) can be a challenging and vulnerable time for infant nutrition due to disproportionately high requirements for metabolic processes, rapid developmental processes, and limited gastric capacity. This is a period of crucial brain development where high caloric intake is necessary to allow synaptogenesis (creation of channels between neurons for communication), and maintenance of established synapses, myelination (laying the myelin sheath around neuronal axons) and everyday psychological functioning. Key nutrients needed for infant brain development include iron (required for oxygen provision to metabolize energy), fatty acids (for cellular membranes and myelin) and protein (for structural support, such as in myelin). Deficiencies in key nutrients during the complementary feeding period have been consistently linked to child development outcomes. Observational studies have consistently demonstrated links between nutrient deficiencies and impairments in intellectual abilities, work capacity, behavioral functioning and even delayed mental and motor development. Yet results from a number of interventions using food, individual nutrients or multiple micronutrients with child development assessments are mixed, possibly partly due to differences in interventions (nutrients and timing), populations, baseline nutrient status, sample sizes, attrition and method of assessment.

Introduction

Complementary feeding is generally the 6- to 24-month period when foods and liquids need to be added to the infant diet to supplement breast milk to ensure nutritional needs are met [1, 2]. However, it can be a time of vulnerability for infants with a high incidence of malnutrition and specific nutrient deficiencies [1].

Six to 24 months is a period of rapid and intense brain development where adequate nutrition is essential to lay the anatomical foundations for normal psychological development. Nutrition is the most influential non-genetic factor affecting early brain development where developmental deficits acquired during infancy due to malnutrition or specific micronutrient deficiencies can be difficult to compensate for later in childhood, even when nutritional status is corrected.

Development of the Infant Brain during the Complementary Feeding Period (6–24 Months)

The complementary feeding period is considered to be one of the critical windows for brain development. The rate of growth is such that a newborn infant brain will grow from 25% of its adult size to 80% by 24 months of age [3]. Early brain development is genetically pre-programmed to occur in a specific order, with intense bursts of developmental processes occurring in specific neurological regions. The two key developmental processes occurring during this time are myelination and synaptogenesis [3]. Neurons (primary brain cells) transmit electrical impulses along an axon to communicate with other neurons [3]. Infants undergo a rapid period of myelination (a myelin sheath created around an axon to speed up the rate an electrical impulse will pass along it) and synaptogenesis (synapses – or connections – between neurons form to allow communication) [3]. During the 6- to 24-month period, synaptogenesis occurs at an astonishingly rapid rate with up to 700 synapses formed per second [3]. Myelination and synaptogenesis increase the rate of information processing and are localized to the areas of the brain necessary for controlling movements (known as motor abilities), language, memory, cognition, and emotion, continually enabling the emergence of new developmental milestones during the 6- to 24-month period [3]. A dependent 6-month-old will grow into an active, mobile toddler capable of eating solids, speaking in two-word sentences and experiencing emotions such as guilt, shame, embarrassment, frustration, possessiveness and excitement in just 18 months [3]. Whilst an individual will continue to develop after 24 months of age, the foundations are laid prior to this time so that early disruptions to development can have long-lasting implications for later outcomes.

Complementary Feeding, Micronutrients, and Infant Brain Development

Early brain development is highly dependent on the timed presence of specific nutrients in sufficient quantities. During the 6- to 24-month period, the brain is undergoing intense myelination and synaptogenesis, both of which require vast

Table 1. Micronutrients in the nervous system

Nutrient	Role	Dietary sources
Protein	Role in cellular structure, components of neurotransmitters and enzymes	Meat and animal products, seafood, legumes, soy
Energy (glucose)	Energy for growth, nerve impulses, synapses	Carbohydrates, such as cereals and grains, fruit
Fatty acids (ω-3/ω-6)	Structural components of cellular membranes as phospholipids, role in neurotransmitter release and neuronal use of glucose	Fish, seafood, meat, poultry, olive oil, nuts, avocado, eggs
Iron	Carries oxygen through the blood stream to be used in the conversion of glucose into energy; component of enzymes needed for neurotransmitters and nervous system stem cell division	Meat and animal products, legumes, spinach, nuts, fortified cereals
Zinc	Role in DNA and RNA synthesis (needed for cell division), component of binding proteins that contribute to neural tissue structure and function, concentrated in hippocampus	Oysters, egg, shellfish, meat, nuts, seeds
Iodine	Needed for making thyroid hormones, which are needed for CNS development (including neurogenesis, neuronal migration, synaptogenesis and myelination)	Marine foods (i.e. fish, shellfish), fortified salt

amounts of energy. Furthermore, established synapses have high energy needs to remain functional so that although the brain is only 2% of the body's mass, it consumes up to 20% of the energy used by the body. Other nutrients considered essential for infant brain development are summarized in table 1. The brain is roughly 10% lipids, such as fatty acids docosahexaenoic acid (DHA: ω-3) DHA, arachidonic acid (ARA: ω-6) and oleic acid (ω-9), as functional components of cellular membranes and 8% protein as the structural support for neural cells and the main component of hormones and chemical signals used for communication between neurons [4]. These key nutrients, along with a variety of others, are in (disproportionately) high demand between 6 and 24 months of age due to rapid brain development in this period.

The caloric and nutritional needs of the infant brain compete with needs of the rest of the body as the infant becomes increasingly active, grows to approximately half of their adult height, and quadruples their birth weight. As growth and development are genetically pre-programmed to occur during this age range, inadequate nutrition will hinder development. Infants are vulnerable to malnutrition and nutrient-specific deficiencies in the complementary feeding period due to their nutritional requirements (from their metabolic rate and rapid development), limited gastric capacity and feeding abilities and lack of access to nutritious complementary foods, such as due to poverty or location, and poor infant feeding practices such as early or late introduction of complementary foods or replacement of breast milk feeds [1].

Whilst global rates for nutritional insufficiency in infancy are currently unknown, 293 million preschool children have anemia, primarily from iron deficiency [5], 101 million are underweight, and 165 million are stunted [6]. Much has been learnt about the effects of deficiencies on brain development from observational studies in populations with endemic deficiency. However, given the concurrence of nutritional deficiencies with other risk factors for suboptimal development such as poor sanitation, education and health care as well as poverty, randomized controlled trials (RCTs) are needed to provide causal evidence. The following is a brief overview of the effects of deficiency and the results of RCTs that have investigated key nutrients during the complementary feeding period and child development (summarized in table 2).

Malnutrition (Calories and Proteins)

Malnutrition can lead to impairments in intellectual abilities, work capacity, behavioral functioning and even delayed mental and motor development [7]. Environmental stimulation has an important role in infant and child development. Malnutrition may also effect child development indirectly through the limiting of physical activity, and feelings of malaise negatively impacting on the infant's experience and interaction with and exploration of the environment. Malnourished children displaying physical symptoms of stunting or underweight underperform in cognitive and motor tasks and academic achievement even in adolescence [7]. A review reported a strong link between childhood malnutrition and lower IQ, poorer cognitive function, lower academic performance and more behavioral problems [8]. Protein deficiency-related malnutrition causes poor growth outcomes and is linked to delayed motor and cognitive development [7]. A series of RCTs has provided protein-, fat- and/or energy-rich food or drinks to whole families, individual infants or day care centers in developing countries in poor communities with prevalent malnutrition [9–14]. Of three trials that assessed early mental development, one reported a benefit of intervention [7], one found no effect [10], and one reported both a benefit and null effect between the two measures used [9]. However, benefits of intervention were found for all motor outcomes [10, 13], infant activity [14], and academic abilities at 11–24 years [12]. A trial specifically targeting only stunted infants found baseline performance below expected levels and improvement after intervention [11] whilst additional fat did not provide greater benefit for observed activity levels compared with just micronutrient supplementation in a population with stunting

Table 2. Nutritional intervention trials in the complementary feeding period (6–23 months) with child development outcomes

First author (year) Location (sample size) Population, diet and nutrient characteristics	Intervention	Outcome assessment and result
Energy/calories/protein		
Waber [9] (1981) Colombia (n = 114) families Population with mild-to-moderate malnutrition Also had intervention group of pregnant women and infants <6 months and group from pregnancy to 36 months	1 Enriched food (bread, dry skim milk, cooking oil, high-protein vegetable mixture) for the whole family, supplements (vitamin A and iron) and maternal education 2 Maternal education (no food) Infants aged 6 months, until 36 months	Griffiths at 6, 12, 24 and 36 months: benefit to mean score across all ages Corman-Escalona Einstein cognitive competence scales at 6, 12, and 18 months: null effect * Tests administered by trained high-school women, not clinicians
Husaini [10] (1991) Indonesia (n = 113) Tea plantation settlements, public bathrooms, low level of parental education	1 Protein and energy snacks provided to day care centers 6 days/week 2 No snacks Infants aged 6–20 months, for 4 months	BSID at baseline and 10–24 months: null effect on mental, but benefit to motor development
Grantham-McGregor [11] (1991) Jamaica (n = 129) Singleton stunted infants in poor neighborhoods, poor housing standard and low level of parental education	1 Powdered formula 2 Stimulation (toys/play time for infant) 3 Powdered formula and stimulation 4 Control (no intervention) 5 Reference group nonstunted children Infants aged 9–24 months, for 2 years	Griffiths every 6 months (from baseline to 24 month): benefit to general development Biggest benefit for powdered formula with stimulation
Pollit [12] (1993) Guatemala, (n = n.r.) Rural villages	1 Calorie and protein-rich drinks 2 Low-calorie drink Infants aged 0–7 years, until they turned 7 years	Benefits to knowledge, numeracy, reading, vocabulary, 11–24 years Biggest benefits for supplementation if commenced before 24 months
Jahari [13] (2000) Indonesia (n = 136) Nutritionally at-risk children	1 High calories with iron 2 Low calories with iron 3 Low calorie Infants aged 12 or 18 months, for 1 year	BSID (motor only) at 24–30 months: benefit to high-calorie with iron Parent-reported motor milestones weekly: benefit to high-calorie with iron
Aburto [14] (2010) Mexico (n = 187) Communities with prevalent micronutrient deficiencies and stunting, but excluded anemia, wasting and chronic disease	1 Micronutrient powder or micronutrient syrup Milk-based 2 fortified food (macronutrients and micronutrients) Infants aged 4–12 months, for 4 months vs. delayed supplementation (infants aged 8–12 months)	Observed physical activity and exploration at 8–16 months: similar benefit to both groups compared with delayed intervention Observed motor development milestones at 8–16 months: n.r.
Fatty acids		
Auestad [17] (2001) United States (n = 404) Healthy, term-born infants	1 DHA and ARA formula (from fish and fungal oil or egg triglycerides) 2 Control formula 3 Nonrandomized breastfed group Infants 0–9 days, for 12 months	Fagan at 6 and 9 months: null effect BSID at 6 and 12 months: null effect MBCDI at 9 and 14 months: null effect Infant Behavior Questionnaire (temperament) at 6 and 12 months: null effect

Table 2. Continued

First author (year) Location (sample size) Population, diet and nutrient characteristics	Intervention	Outcome assessment and result
Drover [18, 19] (2011) United States (n = 181) Healthy, term-born, formula-fed infants, low SES	1 Formula: no DHA or ARA 2 Formula: 0.32% DHA and 0.64% ARA 3 Formula: 0.64% DHA and 0.64% ARA 4 Formula: 0.96% DHA and 0.64% ARA Infants 1–9 days, until 12 months	BSID II at 18 months: groups 2–4 combined benefitted cognition, null effect on motor BSID BRS at 18 months: null effect MBCDI at 18 months: null effect BBCS-R at 25 years: null effect PPVT-III at 2, 35, and 6 years: negative effect on language in DHA and ARA groups at 2 years, null effect at 35 years, benefit at 6 years Executive functioning tasks at 24, 30, 36, 42, 48, 60, and 72 months: null effect on many tasks, benefit to some tasks at 36, 42, 48, and 60 months WPPSI at 7 years: null effect on IQ or performance IQ, but benefit in verbal IQ
Phuka [22] (2012) Malawi (n = 163) Rural community with prevalent stunting	1 50 g micronutrient-fortified lipid spread 2 25 g micronutrient-fortified lipid spread 3 Micronutrient-fortified corn-soy flour Infants aged 6 months, for 12 months	Griffiths at 18 months: null effect
van der Merwe [21] (2013) Gambia (n = 183) Singletons with no HIV only Endemic poor growth and infection, subsistence farming (rice)	1 Fish oil 2 Olive oil Infants aged 3 months, for 6 months	WIPT at 12 months: null effect Attention at 12 months: null effect
Iron		
Lozoff [26] (1982) Guatemala (n = 68) Full-term infants with low and normal hemoglobin levels at baseline Impoverished living conditions (settlement) and low parental education	1 Iron 2 Placebo Infants aged 6–24 months, for 1 week	BSID at baseline and after 1 week (6–24 months): null effect
Aukett [27] (1986) England (n = 97) Inner city but underprivileged anemic infants	1 Iron and vitamin C 2 Vitamin C Infants 17–19 months, for 2 months	DDST (motor) at baseline and 19–21 months: null effect, although more treated children achieved expected development at 19–21 months
Idjradinata [28] (1993) Indonesia (n = 126) Iron-deficient or -sufficient infants, no previous motor delay, stunting or supplement use	1 Iron syrup 2 Placebo syrup Infants aged 12–18 months, for 4 months	BSID at baseline and at 16–22 months: null effect BSID BRS at baseline and at 16–22 months: not reported

Table 2. Continued

First author (year) Location (sample size) Population, diet and nutrient characteristics	Intervention	Outcome assessment and result
Yalcin [29] (2000) Turkey (n = 24) Iron-sufficient infants	1 Iron 2 Placebo Infants 6 months, for 3 months	BSID at 9 months: null effect
Akman [30] (2004) Turkey (n = 108) Singleton, normal birth weight infants, no motor or mental disability, stunting or supplement use, impoverished living conditions, and low parental education	1 Iron 2 No treatment All iron-deficient anemic infants assigned to iron, nonanemic iron-deficient infants assigned to iron or no treatment, iron-sufficient infants not treated Infants aged 6–30 months, for 3 months	BSID at baseline and 6–33 months: null effect DDST at baseline and 6–33 months: null effect
Iodine		
Cao [34] (1994) China (n = 171 aged 12–24 months; n = 170 aged 3–12 months) Endemic severe iodine deficiency, goiter and cretinism, widespread rickets, protein-energy malnutrition and high infant mortality Also supplemented pregnant women, newborns, and older children	1 Iodine (oral oil once every 6 months) 2 Delayed iodine (after outcome assessment) Infants aged 12–24 months	Select BSID test items at 24 months: null effect Physician administered standardized motor assessment every 6 months: null effect Null effect on neurologic outcome at 12–24 months
Trowbridge [35] (1972) Ecuador (n = 35) Endemic severe iodine deficiency, cretinism, and goiter	1 Iodine 2 Comparison group Infants 0–9 months	Stanford-Binet at 3 and 5 years: null effect
Zinc		
Bentley [38] (1997) Guatemala (n = 108) Endemic zinc deficiency and stunting	1 Zinc 2 Placebo Infants aged 6–9 months, for 7 months	Infant activity levels (home observation, including motor milestones) at 9–12 and 13–16 months: null effect to motor milestones, benefit to activity levels at 13–16 months
Gardner [39] (2005) Jamaica, (n = 114) Infants with poor growth, likelihood of baseline zinc deficiency	1 Zinc syrup and micronutrient 2 Stimulation and micronutrient 3 Zinc syrup, stimulation, and micronutrient 4 Micronutrient Infants aged 9–30 months, for 6 months	Griffiths at 0–9 months and 15–36 months: zinc alone benefited 1 subscale, zinc and stimulation benefitted developmental quotient at 15–36 months
Taneja [40] (2005) India, (n = 2,482; 571 with outcome) Endemic zinc deficiency and infection	1 Zinc syrup 2 Placebo syrup Infants aged 6–30 months, for 4 months	BSID II at 12–18 months: null effect

Table 2. Continued

First author (year) Location (sample size) Population, diet and nutrient characteristics	Intervention	Outcome assessment and result
Colombo [41] (2014) Peru (n = 251) Healthy, full-term infants Large shantytown, but access to electricity and water, endemic inadequate calcium, iron, and zinc	1 Liquid zinc, iron, and copper 2 Liquid iron and copper Infants aged 6 months, for 12 months	Visual habituation at 6, 9, and 12 months: some benefit at 9 and 12 months BSID II at 6, 12, and 18 months: null effect Recognition memory at 6, 9, and 12 months: null effect Attention at 12 and 18 months: null effect Spatial working memory task at 9 and 12 months: null effect
Multiple micronutrients		
Black [43] (2004) Bangladesh (n = 221) Rural population of farmers and fishermen with limited access to electricity, safe water, sanitation, low level of parental education High risk of malnutrition, micronutrient deficiencies, and poor diet, but excluded if formula fed, anemic, or severely malnourished	1 Iron liquid 2 Zinc liquid 3 Iron and zinc liquid 4 Multiple micronutrients (including iron and zinc, at 2× RDI) liquid (was not well tolerated, many vomited afterwards) 5 Riboflavin (control) liquid Infants aged 6 months, for 6 months	BSID II at baseline and 12 months: all motor scores were lower after intervention, but lowest in the control group; mental development: n.r. BSID BRS at baseline and 12 months: n.r., except for exploration score (benefited from any intervention)
Lind [44] (2004) Indonesia (n = 680) Population with prevalent child malnutrition, stunting, and micronutrient deficiencies Healthy singletons, excluding anemia	1 Zinc syrup 2 Iron syrup 3 Zinc and iron syrup 4 Placebo syrup (vomiting after ingestion reported in groups 1 and 3) Infants aged 6 months, until 12 months	BSID at baseline and 12 months: iron benefitted motor development but iron with zinc had null effect, mental Development: n.r. BSID BRS at baseline and 12 months: n.r.
Faber [45] (2005) South Africa (n = 361) Rural low SES area with low population density, low malnutrition but endemic micronutrient deficiency	1 Fortified (iron, zinc, copper, selenium, and vitamins B, E, A) porridge 2 Unfortified porridge Infants aged 6–12 months, for 6 months	Parent-reported motor milestones at 12–18 months: benefit to motor development
Wang [46] (2006) Chen [50] (2010) China (n = 1,478) Rural low SES villages Breastfed infants	1 Infant formula and sachet to add to complimentary food (soybean flour with 5 micronutrients), and vitamin A supplement every 6 months 2 Infant formula and sachet to add to complimentary food (rice flour, no micronutrients, and low protein), and vitamin A supplement every 6 months 3 Control children from another village Infants 4–12 months, until 24 months	Developmental diagnostic scale at 24 months: benefit to overall quotient for group 1 and 2, benefit to motor development for group 1, null effect on language and behavior Developmental diagnostic scale at 3.5–4 and 4.5–5 years: benefit to overall quotient for group 1 and 2 at 3.5–4 years but null effect at 4.5–5 years WPPSI at 5.5–6 years: benefit for group 1

Table 2. Continued

First author (year) Location (sample size) Population, diet and nutrient characteristics	Intervention	Outcome assessment and result
Adu-Afarwuah [47] (2007) Ghana (n = 313) Breastfed infants	1 6 micronutrients in a sprinkles sachet (iron + zinc) 2 16 micronutrients in a crushable tablet (iron, zinc, and iodine) 3 19 micronutrients in a lipid spread (iron, zinc, iodine, and fatty acids) 4 No intervention (enrolled at 12 months) Infants aged 6 months, until 12 months	4 motor milestones at 12 months: all interventions increased likelihood of walking independently at 12 months
Katz [48] (2010) Surkan [49] (2013) Nepal (n = 3,264) Rural villages, common micronutrient deficiencies	1 Iron and folic acid tablet 2 Zinc tablet 3 Iron, folic acid, and zinc tablet 4 Placebo tablet Infants aged 1–35 months, until they reached 36 months	Parent-reported motor milestones at 4–17 months: null effect Parent-reported language milestones at 4–17 months: null effect

BBCS-R = Bracken Basic Concept Scale – Revised: school readiness; BSID = Bayley Scales of Infant Development (version I or II) – standardized mental (cognitive) and motor development scales; BSID BRS = Bayley Scales of Infant Development (version I or II) Behavior Rating Scale – behavior; DDST = Denver Developmental Screening Test – 24 motor items only; Fagan = Fagan Test of Infant Intelligence – novelty preference (information processing); Griffiths = Griffiths Mental Development Scale – standardized global development; IQ = intelligence quotient; MBCDI = MacArthur Communicative Development Inventories; parent-reported standardized language development; n.r. = not reported; PPVT-III = Peabody Picture Vocabulary Test – 3rd edition; standardized language development; SES = socioeconomic status; Stanford-Binet = Stanford-Binet Intelligence Scales – standardized intelligence (cognitive ability); WIPT = Willats' Infant Planning Test – problem solving; WPPSI = Wechsler Primary Preschool Scale of Intelligence – standardized IQ (cognition).

and micronutrient deficiencies [14]. However, as pointed out by several authors, food provided to families for infants may have been consumed by other family members. Interestingly, two studies with long intervention periods reported the most benefits from intervention during the complementary feeding period, rather than supplementation during pregnancy and the first 6 months of life [9] or after 24 months of age [12].

Fatty Acids

The fatty acids DHA and ARA have important structural roles within the brain, particularly within the cellular membrane phospholipid layer due to their functional structure [15]. Meta-analyses of infant formula trials have not shown an improvement in developmental outcomes of full-term infants given or not given DHA and/or ARA [16]. Whilst the majority of RCTs ceased intervention at

4–6 months of age, two trials that continued formula intervention to 12 months had mixed results; one found a null effect on temperament and mental, motor and language development [17], and the other found null effects on the majority of outcomes including behavior, motor development and IQ, but possible positive effects on early mental development and some experimental executive function tasks, a negative effect in one language assessment and a benefit in a later language assessment [18–20]. Both of these trials were conducted in healthy, full-term infants in a developed country (the United States). The only non-formula fatty acid interventions during the complementary feeding period found no benefit of fish oil (rich in DHA) over olive oil for problem solving or attention [21] and no benefit of fatty acid spread over a corn-soy flour for general development, although both groups received micronutrients [22]. Three of these trials commenced intervention before 6 months of age [17, 18, 21], and were either in developed countries [17, 18] or populations where children were likely to be replete with fatty acids [21, 22], so the effect of fatty acid supplementation during the complementary feeding period is unclear. Preterm infants, who missed the full gestational supply of fatty acids and are likely to have received suboptimal amounts, tend to show benefit from infant formulas containing DHA and/or ARA, but again the majority of these trials stop intervention prior to 6 months of age [23].

Iron

Iron is needed for the synthesis of hemoglobin, which carries oxygen from the lungs around the body through the bloodstream to be used by various tissues in the conversion of glucose into energy. Iron deficiency results in reduced oxygen-carrying capacity, which in turn will limit the conversion of the glucose needed for growth and development. The brain has a high glucose requirement, which relies on adequate iron as it uses 20% of the body's oxygen. Additionally, nervous system development relies on iron-containing proteins and enzymes, such as those necessary for signal controlling in some neurotransmitters (including dopamine and serotonin). Initially, infants rely on iron liver reserves built up during pregnancy, as iron content of breast milk is low [1]. By around 6 months, these stores deplete and complementary foods must provide iron requirements from this time onwards [24]. Meat is the best source of bioavailable iron; however, even in developed countries where meat is readily available, many infants are considered iron deficient and iron-fortified infant cereals are a more prevalent dietary source of iron [25].

The combination of high iron requirements between 6 and 24 months and problematic dietary supply contributes to high rates of iron deficiency internationally [5]. Because of widespread iron deficiency in infancy and the detrimental effects on development, the World Health Organization recommends daily iron supplementation for all children aged 6–24 months if the diet does not include food fortified with iron [25].

A review of observational studies links iron deficiency anemia prior to 24 months to increased risk of poor cognitive, motor, social-emotional, language, behavioral, and neurophysiologic development as well as a 6- to 15-point drop in developmental test scores compared to iron-sufficient infants with deficits in cognition and school achievement lasting into adolescence [24]. RCTs of iron supplementation in the complementary feeding period have generally reported no difference between iron and control supplements on cognitive or motor development [26–30]. All but one trial included iron-deficient children [29]. Three trials reported that iron-deficient children scored well below iron-sufficient children prior to supplementation but caught up by the end of the intervention [27, 28, 30]. One trial reported no improvement in mental or motor development after supplementation to infants with low hemoglobin levels; however, given the small sample and short intervention period (6–8 days) [26], it is possible that infants with mild deficits due to iron deficiency could recover if iron is restored.

Iodine

Iodine is necessary for synthesizing thyroid hormones, which are needed for nervous system development processes such as synaptogenesis and myelination. After birth, iodine deficiency can cause thyroid failure, which may lead to hypothyroidism. A meta-analysis of observational studies showed that individuals who lived in iodine-deficient areas scored 13.5 IQ points lower than individuals in iodine-sufficient areas [31]. Although many countries now have iodized salt widely available, mild-to-moderate iodine deficiency is still a concern in many developed and developing countries. Iodine intervention studies have largely targeted pregnant women [32, 33], with a few studies correcting iodine deficiency in infants shortly after birth or after 2 years of age [33]. Two studies that included supplementation during the complementary feeding period in populations with prevalent iodine deficiency found no benefit for cognitive development [34, 35]. This contrasts with a review of non-randomized interventions in children under 6 years of age showing a difference of 6.9–8.1 IQ points between iodine and placebo groups [33] but is in line with interventions during pregnancy [32, 36]. Iodine intervention before or during pregnancy seems to lower the risk of cretinism, yet the effects on child cognitive and motor development have been unclear with reports of benefits, null effects and even negative effects [32, 36].

Zinc

Zinc has a role in numerous processes with implications for brain development such as a component of enzymes needed for the synthesis and metabolism of carbohydrates, lipids and proteins as well as other micronutrient metabolism [37]. Zinc is the fourth most abundant ion in the brain as a component of the binding proteins that contribute to structure and function [37]. Four trials of zinc supplementation that were inclusive of the complementary feeding period found mainly null effects on mental and motor development [38–41]. However, two trials reported some evidence of benefit on non-standardised or robust measures [38, 41], and another stated that zinc combined with stimulation increased the developmental quotient [39]. All trials were conducted in developing countries with widespread zinc deficiency, but there was no difference in effect for infants who were or were not stunted at baseline [38]. The effect of zinc supplementation during the 6- to 24-month period on child development is still unclear, a finding which supports meta-analyses of zinc interventions throughout childhood with developmental outcomes [42].

Multiple Micronutrients

Micronutrient deficiencies often co-occur, particularly in impoverished areas, so that a single micronutrient supplement may be insufficient to improve outcomes. RCTs intervening with multiple micronutrients in developing countries during the complementary feeding period consistently included zinc and iron, with or without other nutrients across multiple intervention groups [43–49]. One trial that assessed mental development yearly between 2 and 6 years of age consistently found higher scores in supplemented children [46, 50] whilst two other studies did not report the results of the mental development score of the Bayley Scales of Infant Development [43, 44]. Four trials found benefits to motor development in one [44, 46] or all variations of intervention [45, 47]; however, one trial found a decrease in motor scores in all children after the 6-month intervention period [43]. Two trials with language outcomes reported no difference in scores according to intervention group [46, 48, 49]. Results of multiple micronutrient interventions did not appear to differ according to whether intervention was supplied as a tablet or in food (such as porridge or formula) although two studies reported low tolerance and vomiting after ingestion of some liquid and syrup supplements [43, 44] with increased stunting and wasting after the intervention in one trial [44]. Effects of multiple micronutrient interventions in the complementary period on child development are currently unclear, in agreement with a recent Cochrane review of multiple micronutrient powders during this period for numerous outcomes that reported convincing benefits only for reducing iron deficiency [51].

Summary and Conclusion

Despite observational studies consistently linking infant nutritional deficiencies with deficits in child development (particularly cognition), RCTs of nutritional interventions during the complementary feeding period have been less convincing. As observational studies are unable to establish causality, it is possible that other confounding factors are driving the association. Much of the observational studies are in poor communities where nutritional quality, sanitation and parental education is poor, and multiple micronutrient deficiencies are likely. In such situations, intervention with nutrition only is unlikely to correct for all contributions to suboptimal development. Additionally, many of the studies experienced difficulties in ensuring infants consumed the administered intervention; one trial provided surplus formula with the presumption that it would be shared amongst family members [11] while others provided food for the whole family [9], or to day care centers [10] or had study staff visit families every day to administer intervention [26, 38]. Furthermore, nutritional RCTs during the complementary feeding period are generally designed to investigate non-developmental outcomes. As reported by two recent Cochrane reviews of multiple micronutrient powders for infants [51] and food in childhood [52], there are many nutritional trials that do not assess cognitive or motor development. Furthermore, early global assessments used by many studies, such as the Bayley Scales of Infant Development, are not considered ideal for assessing effects of nutrition on mental development [53]. Other issues prevalent in some of these RCTs are quasi-randomization and clustering, lack of blinding (particularly when controls received no intervention) and high attrition. Given the significance of development during the 6- to 24-month period for later health outcomes, public national and international health policies to improve infant nutrition may be an effective means of improving general population health. However, the current evidence base highlights the need for future large, quality RCTs of specific nutrients to determine how best to promote optimal development.

Disclosure Statement

J.F.G. received honoraria (payable to her institution) from the Nestlé Nutrition Institute. Honoraria will be used to support conference travel.

References

1 World Health Organization: Guiding Principles for Complementary Feeding of the Breastfed Child. World Health Organization, 2003.

2 World Health Organization: Infant and Young Child Feeding. Geneva, World Health Organization, 2016, Fact sheet 342.

3 Hoffnung M, Hoffnung RJ, Seifert KL, et al: Lifespan Development: A Chronological Approach, 2nd Australasian Edition. Milton, Wiley, 2013.

4 McIlwain H, Bachelard HS: Biochemistry and the Central Nervous System. Edinburgh, Churchill Livingstone, 1985.

5 World Health Organization: Centers for Disease Control and Prevention: Worldwide Prevalence of Anaemia 1993–2005. WHO Global Database on Anaemia. Geneva, World Health Organization, 2008.

6 Black RE, Allen LH, Bhutta ZA, et al: Maternal and child undernutrition: global and regional exposures and health consequences. Lancet 2008;371:243–260.

7 Grantham-McGregor S, Baker-Henningham H: Review of the evidence linking protein and energy to mental development. Public Health Nutr 2005;8:1191–1201.

8 Grantham-McGregor S: A review of studies of the effect of severe malnutrition on mental development. J Nutr 1995;125(suppl):2233S–2238S.

9 Waber DP, Vuori-Christiansen L, Ortiz N, et al: Nutritional supplementation, maternal education, and cognitive development of infants at risk of malnutrition. Am J Clin Nutr 1981;34(suppl 4):807–813.

10 Husaini MA, Karyadi L, Husaini YK, et al: Developmental effects of short-term supplementary feeding in nutritionally-at-risk Indonesian infants. Am J Clin Nutr 1991;54:799–804.

11 Grantham-McGregor SM, Powell CA, Walker SP, et al: Nutritional supplementation, psychosocial stimulation, and mental development of stunted children: the Jamaican Study. Lancet 1991;338:1–5.

12 Pollitt E, Gorman KS, Engle PL, et al: Early supplementary feeding and cognition: effects over two decades. Monogr Soc Res Child Dev 1993;58:1–99; discussion 111–118.

13 Jahari AB, Saco-Pollitt C, Husaini MA, et al: Effects of an energy and micronutrient supplement on motor development and motor activity in undernourished children in Indonesia. Eur J Clin Nutr 2000;54(suppl 2):S60–S68.

14 Aburto NJ, Ramirez-Zea M, Neufeld LM, et al: The effect of nutritional supplementation on physical activity and exploratory behavior of Mexican infants aged 8–12 months. Eur J Clin Nutr 2010;64:644–651.

15 Uauy R, Dangour AD: Nutrition in brain development and aging: role of essential fatty acids. Nutr Rev 2006;64:S24–S33; discussion S72–S91.

16 Simmer K, Patole SK, Rao SC: Long-chain polyunsaturated fatty acid supplementation in infants born at term. Cochrane Database Syst Rev 2011;12:CD000376.

17 Auestad N, Halter R, Hall RT, et al: Growth and development in term infants fed long-chain polyunsaturated fatty acids: a double-masked, randomized, parallel, prospective, multivariate study. Pediatrics 2001;108:372–381.

18 Drover JR, Hoffman DR, Castañeda YS, et al: Cognitive function in 18-month-old term infants of the DIAMOND study: a randomized, controlled clinical trial with multiple dietary levels of docosahexaenoic acid. Early Hum Dev 2011;87:223–230.

19 Drover JR, Felius J, Hoffman DR, et al: A randomized trial of DHA intake during infancy: school readiness and receptive vocabulary at 2–3.5 years of age. Early Hum Dev 2012;88: 885–891.

20 Colombo J, Carlson SE, Cheatham CL, et al: Long-term effects of LCPUFA supplementation on childhood cognitive outcomes. Am J Clin Nutr 2013;98:403–412.

21 van der Merwe LF, Moore SE, Fulford AJ, et al: Long-chain PUFA supplementation in rural African infants: a randomized controlled trial of effects on gut integrity, growth, and cognitive development. Am J Clin Nutr 2013;97:45–57.

22 Phuka JC, Gladstone M, Maleta K, et al: Developmental outcomes among 18-month-old Malawians after a year of complementary feeding with lipid-based nutrient supplements or corn-soy flour. Matern Child Nutr 2012;8:239–248.

23 Schulzke SM, Patole SK, Simmer K: Long-chain polyunsaturated fatty acid supplementation in preterm infants. Cochrane Database Syst Rev 2011;2:CD000375.
24 Lozoff B, Beard J, Connor J, et al: Long-lasting neural and behavioral effects of iron deficiency in infancy. Nutr Rev 2006;64:S34–S43; discussion S72–S91.
25 World Health Organisation: Essential Nutrition Actions: Improving Maternal, Newborn, Infant and Young Child Health and Nutrition. Geneva, WHO, 2013.
26 Lozoff B, Brittenham GM, Viteri FE, et al: The effects of short-term oral iron therapy on developmental deficits in iron-deficient anemic infants. J Pediatr 1982;100:351–357.
27 Aukett MA, Parks YA, Scott PH, et al: Treatment with iron increases weight gain and psychomotor development. Arch Dis Childhood 1986;61:849–857.
28 Idjradinata P, Pollitt E: Reversal of developmental delays in iron-deficient anaemic infants treated with iron. Lancet 1993;341:1–4.
29 Yalcin SS, Yurdakok K, Acikgoz D, et al: Short-term developmental outcome of iron prophylaxis in infants. Pediatr Int 2000;42:625–630.
30 Akman M, Cebeci D, Okur V, et al: The effects of iron deficiency on infants' developmental test performance. Acta Paediatr 2004;93:1391–1396.
31 Blelchrodt N, Born M: A metaanalysis of research on iodine and its relationship to cognitive development; in Stanbury J (ed): The Damaged Brain of Iodine Deficiency. New York, Cognizant Communication Corporation, 1994, pp 195–200.
32 Zimmermann MB: The effects of iodine deficiency in pregnancy and infancy. Paediatr Perinat Epidemiol 2012;26(suppl 1):108–117.
33 Bougma K, Aboud FE, Harding KB, et al: Iodine and mental development of children 5 years old and under: a systematic review and meta-analysis. Nutrients 2013;5:1384–1416.
34 Cao XY, Jiang XM, Dou ZH, et al: Timing of vulnerability of the brain to iodine deficiency in endemic cretinism. N Engl J Med 1994;331:1739–1744.
35 Trowbridge FL: Intellectual assessment in primitive societies, with a preliminary report of a study of the effects of early iodine supplementation on intelligence. Adv Exp Med Biol 1972;30:137–149.
36 Zhou SJ, Anderson AJ, Gibson RA, et al: Effect of iodine supplementation in pregnancy on child development and other clinical outcomes: a systematic review of randomized controlled trials. Am J Clin Nutr 2013;98:1241–1254.
37 Black MM: Zinc deficiency and child development. Am J Clin Nutr 1998;68(suppl):464S–469S.
38 Bentley ME, Caulfield LE, Ram M, et al: Zinc supplementation affects the activity patterns of rural Guatemalan infants. J Nutr 1997;127:1333–1338.
39 Gardner JM, Powell CA, Baker-Henningham H, et al: Zinc supplementation and psychosocial stimulation: effects on the development of undernourished Jamaican children. Am J Clin Nutr 2005;82:399–405.
40 Taneja S, Bhandari N, Bahl R, et al: Impact of zinc supplementation on mental and psychomotor scores of children aged 12 to 18 months: a randomized, double-blind trial. J Pediatr 2005;146:506–511.
41 Colombo J, Zavaleta N, Kannass KN, et al: Zinc supplementation sustained normative neurodevelopment in a randomized, controlled trial of Peruvian infants aged 6–18 months. J Nutr 2014;144:1298–1305.
42 Brown KH, Peerson JM, Baker SK, et al: Preventive zinc supplementation among infants, preschoolers, and older prepubertal children. Food Nutr Bull 2009;30(suppl):S12–S40.
43 Black MM, Baqui AH, Zaman K, et al: Iron and zinc supplementation promote motor development and exploratory behavior among Bangladeshi infants. Am J Clin Nutr 2004;80:903–910.
44 Lind T, Lonnerdal B, Stenlund H, et al: A community-based randomized controlled trial of iron and zinc supplementation in Indonesian infants: effects on growth and development. Am J Clin Nutr 2004;80:729–736.
45 Faber M, Kvalsvig JD, Lombard CJ, et al: Effect of a fortified maize-meal porridge on anemia, micronutrient status, and motor development of infants. Am J Clin Nutr 2005;82:1032–1039.
46 Wang YY, Wang FZ, Wang K, et al: Effects of nutrient fortified complementary food supplements on development of infants and young children in poor rural area of Gansu Province (in Chinese). Wei Sheng Yan Jiu 2006;35:772–774.

47 Adu-Afarwuah S, Lartey A, Brown KH, et al: Randomized comparison of 3 types of micronutrient supplements for home fortification of complementary foods in Ghana: effects on growth and motor development. Am J Clin Nutr 2007;86:412–420.
48 Katz J, Khatry SK, Leclerq SC, et al: Daily supplementation with iron plus folic acid, zinc, and their combination is not associated with younger age at first walking unassisted in malnourished preschool children from a deficient population in rural Nepal. J Nutr 2010;140:1317–1321.
49 Surkan PJ, Siegel EH, Patel SA, et al: Effects of zinc and iron supplementation fail to improve motor and language milestone scores of infants and toddlers. Nutrition 2013;29: 542–548.
50 Chen CM, Wang YY, Chang SY: Effect of in-home fortification of complementary feeding on intellectual development of Chinese children. Biomed Environ Sci 2010;23:83–91.
51 De-Regil LM, Suchdev PS, Vist GE, et al: Home fortification of foods with multiple micronutrient powders for health and nutrition in children under two years of age (review). Evid Based Child Health 2013;8:112–201.
52 Kristjansson E, Francis DK, Liberato S, et al: Food supplementation for improving the physical and psychosocial health of socio-economically disadvantaged children aged three months to five years. Cochrane Database Syst Rev 2015;3:CD009924.
53 Wainwright PE, Colombo J: Nutrition and the development of cognitive functions: interpretation of behavioral studies in animals and human infants. Am J Clin Nutr 2006;84: 961–970.

Black RE, Makrides M, Ong KK (eds): Complementary Feeding: Building the Foundations for a Healthy Life. Nestlé Nutr Inst Workshop Ser, vol 87, pp 29–38, (DOI: 10.1159/000448935)
Nestec Ltd., Vevey/S. Karger AG., Basel, © 2017

Advancement in Texture in Early Complementary Feeding and the Relevance to Developmental Outcomes

Jordan R. Green[a] · Meg Simione[a] · Benjamin Le Révérend[b] · Erin M. Wilson[c] · Brian Richburg[a] · Marc Alder[b] · Mirna Del Valle[b] · Chrystel Loret[b]

[a]Speech and Feeding Disorders Lab, MGH Institute of Health Professions, Boston, MA, USA; [b]Nestlé Research Center, Lausanne, Switzerland; [c]Waisman Center, University of Madison-Wisconsin, Madison, WI, USA

Abstract

A child's transition to independent eating is a protracted process that progresses over the course of many years. Although major health agencies, such as the World Health Organization, now offer clear guidance when to begin introducing solids, advice about how to safely transition to progressively challenging foods is varied and comes from a staggering number of sources. The resulting conflicting views have promoted parental confusion and anxiety about what foods are appropriate and when to advance to new textures. Efforts to develop science-based recommendations for complementary feeding include research on the development of chewing motor skills. Chewing development is an essential aspect of feeding readiness that is often overlooked by agencies developing recommendations for complementary feeding, and little is known about the development of chewing motor skills and how children learn to accommodate foods with varying textures. Such information is essential for designing developmentally appropriate foods, minimizing food aversions, providing caregivers science-based guidance regarding the safety and appropriateness of new foods, and identifying children at risk for choking or feeding impairments.

Guidelines for Texture Advancement

A child's transition to independent eating is a protracted process that progresses over the course of many years. One particularly difficult decision faced by all parents is when and how best to introduce new, more challenging foods.

Common parental concerns include risks of choking, allergies, nutrition and food refusal/neophobia. Guidance on how to safely transition from soft to hard foods are currently underspecified and come from a variety of sources, which has led to confusion about what foods are appropriate and when to advance to new textures [1, 2].

Major health organizations, such as the World Health Organization, have recently advised delaying the introduction of complementary foods until 6 months of age [1]. When solids are introduced too early, it increases the risk of choking, picky eating, food hypersensitivity, sudden infant death syndrome, and chronic diseases such as diabetes, obesity, asthma, and celiac disease [3]. Alternatively, when solids are introduced too late, a child may not learn to eat solid foods properly, become malnourished, develop iron-deficiency anemia, and not follow the normal growth curve [1, 2]. Despite these known risks, however, many children are being offered solids too early [3] while some are being offered them too late (with some parental-led movements now advocating for delaying solids until after 12 months of age). The emerging research on the importance of not offering solids too soon or too late underscores the delicate balance in pediatric feeding between providing textures that are challenging but safe.

The pace of complementary feeding is typically determined by a variety of factors including sensorimotor development, cultural standards, available resources, and parental decisions based on their child's perceived readiness. A major challenge to developing universal timelines for complementary feeding is the significant differences across families and cultures in preferences regarding the types of foods offered to infants and the advancement of textures. For example, in Europe, North European countries such as Finland and Norway introduced solid foods much earlier than South European countries such as Spain [4]. Another major challenge is the well-known differences among children in their rates of development. For this reason, many guidelines promote the conventional wisdom that food textures should be gradually upgraded based on infants' abilities. The American Academy of Pediatrics [5], for example, suggests that babies should not be fed solids until they reach several key developmental milestones including the doubling of their birth weight, adequate independent control of the neck and head, ability to sit up with minimal support, and ability to refuse food by pulling away or shutting the mouth.

A critical omission from this list is the child's oromotor readiness, that is, the child's ability to efficiently and safely chew and swallow a given texture. Yet, choking due to immature chewing and swallowing skills are the leading causes of morbidity and mortality among children under the age of 3 years (Committee on Injury, Violence, and Poison Prevention [6]). To promote prevention and public awareness of the hazards of food choking, the Food Choking Prevention

Act was introduced in United States Congress three different times between 2002 and 2006 (but unfortunately was never enacted). A likely explanation for the absence of oromotor milestones in current guidelines is the paucity of knowledge about the development of oromotor skills such as chewing. Essential questions that need to be addressed are (1) how can a child's readiness for texture upgrades be determined and (2) what are the texture properties that are appropriate at each phase of chewing development.

From a motor development perspective, a child's readiness for a given food will depend on the match between the developmental status of his/her oromotor system and the demands required to macerate and safely transport the food into the esophagus. Optimal foods will be appropriately adapted to chewing ability, swallowed safely, and provide pleasant early feeding experiences. To address the question of oromotor readiness, a relatively small number of researchers have investigated the development of chewing biomechanics [7–10], which provide a window into oromotor readiness. Chewing is an important component of oromotor development that determines feeding competence and has a surprising number of significant implications for growth, nutrition, safety, and overall well-being. The goals of this research are to improve our understanding of (1) the development of chewing motor skills, (2) the factors that influence chewing development such as the emergence of dentition, and (3) the interaction between a child's oromotor readiness and the physical properties of the food. This information is essential for providing caregivers science-based guidance regarding the safety and appropriateness of new foods, identifying children at risk for choking or feeding impairments, designing new developmentally appropriate foods, and redesigning foods that pose a high risk [11].

The Human Food Processor: The Role of Chewing in Ingestion

Chewing is a lot of work. The average person chews at a rate of roughly 60 times per minute, with an estimated total of 2,700 chews per day, or roughly one million cycles per year. The jaw muscles are among the strongest muscles in the human body with an average maximum male bite force at the molars of approximately 777 N (175 lb). The primary function of chewing is to reduce solids into a cohesive bolus that is mixed with saliva in preparation for swallowing. The breakdown of food through chewing is also essential for facilitating digestion, releasing of essential nutrients [12], and triggering satiety. Chewing also makes the experience of eating more pleasurable by enhancing textures, taste, and smell. Chewing has at least three sequential stages: cutting, maceration, and transport [13]. During cutting, jaw force is generated to fractionate the food into chewable-sized pieces. During maceration, the bolus is further broken down by the molars while being continuously transported toward the pharynx by the tongue and cheeks. During the transport stage, the tongue helps to form the food into a cohesive bolus that is propelled toward the pharynx using a highly coordinated contractile wave [10]. This decomposition of chewing into its component parts underscores that is a complex skill, dependent on learned sensorimotor experiences.

Why Texture Matters: Chewing Solids for Growth and Development

Although postponing the introduction of solids in the diet until after 6 months of age is clearly an imperative, the timely exposure to solids is essential for promoting the normal development of chewing anatomy, physiology, and neural circuitry. Mastication of solid food generates the levels of muscular loading required to stimulate craniofacial growth and muscle development. Animals reared on soft diets have altered mandibular bone and cartilage growth [14, 15], masticatory muscle weakness [16], improper eruption of permanent teeth, and reduced space in the oral cavity for permanent dentition [17]. Harder foods also provide a rich supply of sensory information from muscle spindles and periodontal mechanoreceptors that modifies the masticatory central pattern generator output. Soft foods, in contrast, do not provide the necessary stimulus for developing supportive neural circuitry [18].

One important question is – if solids are delayed, can a child catch up? The data by Fujishita et al. [18] suggest that normal chewing function, as determined by the number of chewing cycles and chewing biomechanics, is never achieved in mice whose transition to solids is delayed. These findings raise the possibility that masticatory function may never normalize if hard textures are not introduced into the diet at a yet to be determined young age. A delay in solids may also increase the likelihood of rejection of solids later in life [19–22] and the longer the delay, the more difficult it is for many children to accept texture changes [23, 24]. Because children establish dietary preferences and habits in early childhood, aversions to solids may have an enduring impact on health [25].

Chewing as a Learned Sensorimotor Behavior

During the first few years of life, when motor coordination is immature and when many deciduous teeth have yet to emerge, learning to chew poses a significant motor challenge to the young child. Regardless of when challenging

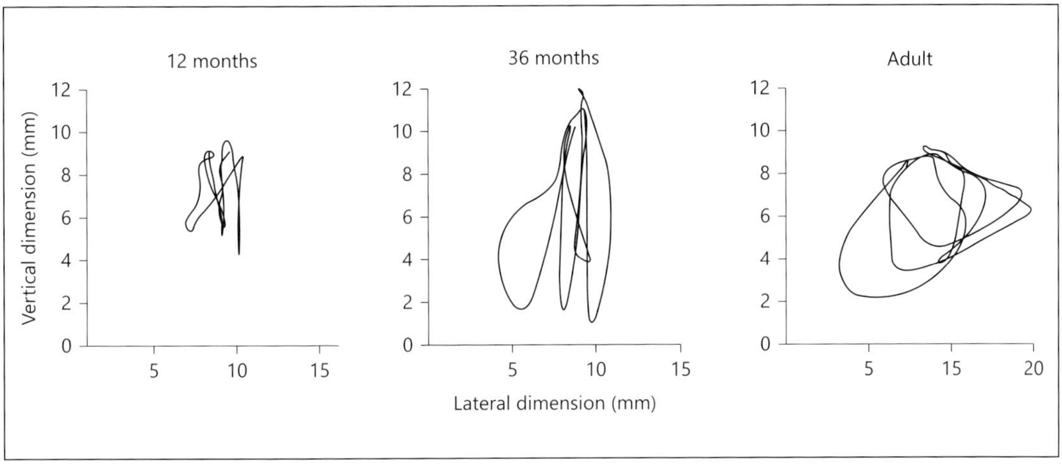

Fig. 1. Example jaw movement trajectories during chewing recorded from a 12-month-old, a 36-month-old, and an adult. With age, jaw motion became more stable, and the occlusal point was more consistent as children progressed from beginning to advanced chewers. Between 12 and 36 months, the vertical displacement of the jaw increased.

textures are introduced, chewing – like other motor behaviors – is learned through an iterative process and is dependent upon anatomic growth, neural maturation, and considerable experience. Chewing motor immaturity is best understood in the context of mature chewing motor skills.

Mature chewing is characterized by rhythmic oscillations of the jaw that are driven by a consistent pattern of reciprocal activation among jaw depressor and elevator muscles. Biomechanical efficiency in the adult chewing pattern is evidenced by highly synchronized activation of the jaw elevator synergists and by the unopposed activation of antagonists during the opening and closing phase of the chewing cycle. Mature chewers are particularly skilled at exploiting elastic (vs. active) muscular forces in order to minimize the work of chewing [7]. Central motor programs stored in the masticatory central pattern generator generate coordinated patterns of jaw muscle activation during chewing (fig. 1) [26, 27]. This pattern is continuously modulated by sensory feedback from intraoral receptors.

Experienced chewers are particularly adept at adapting their chewing patterns depending on the shape, size, and texture of the food. For example, increased food hardness elicits faster jaw movements, greater bite force, larger lateral excursions, and an increase in the number of chews per bite [28]. These adaptations are not only driven by rapid peripheral reflexes (i.e., digastric reflex) mediated by periodontal mechanoreceptors, but also by knowledge of the requirements of the chewing task [29]. Such knowledge may incorporate the large number of sensory cues associated with various foods, including shape, size, surface texture, consistency, flavor, temperature, specific gravity, and granularity. Therefore, children should be exposed to a variety of textures during weaning to be able to recognize these cues and adapt their chewing behavior to the food texture.

In contrast, immature chewing is characterized by significant temporal asynchrony among the activation of synergistic muscles that elevate the jaw as well as increased levels of co-contraction among the jaw antagonistic muscles [8]. In comparison to mature chewing, other documented inefficiencies include increased lateral jaw displacement, prolonged chewing time, and increased number of chewing cycles per sequence [10, 30]. Overall, these findings suggest that although the basic coordinative organization for chewing (i.e., the ability to reciprocally activate jaw elevators and depressors to open and close the mandible) is established in early infancy, chewing skills are refined considerably over many years [8, 10].

Chewing Skills as Physiologic Indicators of Readiness for Different Textures

Our research group is now using biomechanic analyses to test the age appropriateness of solid foods that vary in texture. To accomplish these goals, we are investigating how chewing motor performance in children aged 9–36 months is affected by solid foods with varying textures and by the emergence of molars. Both electromyography and 3D optical motion capture are used to obtain a comprehensive account of masticatory muscle coordination and control (fig. 2). Electromyography can be used to study the underlying coordinative organization of masticatory muscles, such as the emergence and refinement of the temporal coordination and spatial symmetry of synergistic and antagonistic muscle pairs [8]. Optical motion capture, a technology that uses infrared light to track reflective markers in three dimensions, can be used to study fast and subtle facial movements. The research framework is based on the underlying assumption that solid textures that show little change across ages are easy to chew for even inexperienced chewers.

Two age-appropriate, commercial solid food products were tested at each age: Cheerios (General Mills), an oat-based cereal, and Rice Rusks (Hipp), a puffed rice-based cracker. Both products were cut to approximately the same size and volume, and children had been previously exposed to the foods prior to the study. Significant age- and product-related changes were observed from 9 to 36 months as our participants progressed from beginning to more advanced

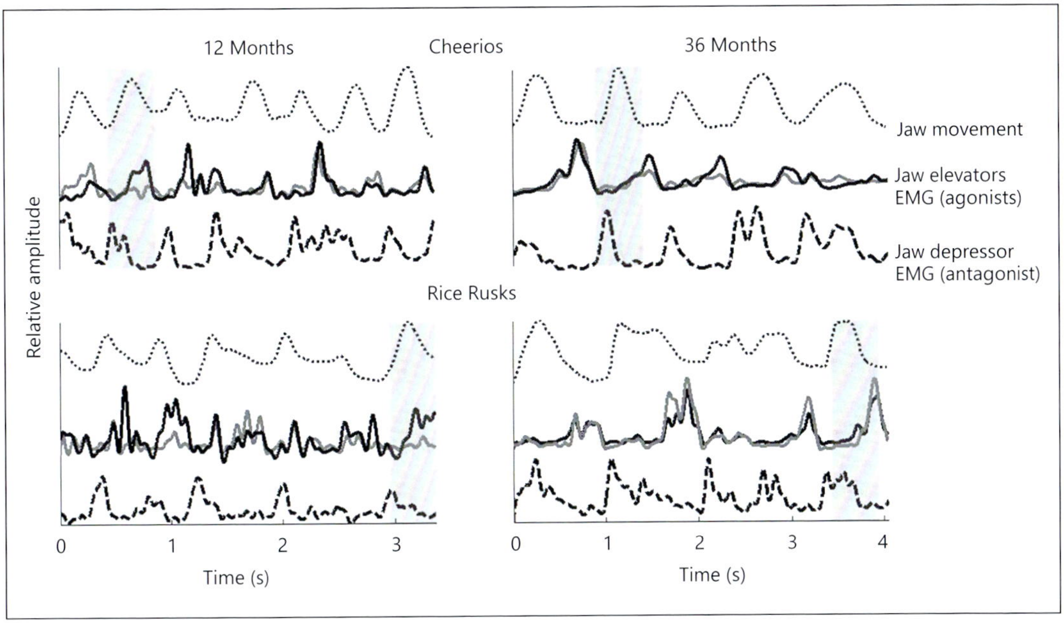

Fig. 2. Kinematic recordings of jaw displacement and activation patterns of synergistic (i.e., jaw elevators) and antagonistic (i.e., jaw depressors) muscles during chewing. The highlighted chewing cycles illustrate that with age chewing cycles became more clearly defined. Also with age, the synergistic muscle pairs became more tightly coupled. In the beginning phases, antagonistic cocontraction was observed, whereas a reciprocal activation pattern predominated for the 36-month-olds. For both ages, a more mature chewing pattern was noted for the Cheerios than the Rice Rusks, suggesting Rice Rusks was mechanically challenging for beginning chewers.

chewers, although 36-month-olds were still not demonstrating adult-like chewing patterns (fig. 3). Chewing behavior varied among the two foods, suggesting that their differing structural properties uniquely affected their mandibular coordination and control. Overall, a more mature chewing pattern (as described in the previous paragraph) was observed for the Cheerios than for the Rice Rusks, suggesting that Rice Rusks biscuits were mechanically challenging for beginning chewers.

In addition, the emergence of teeth was associated with increased synergistic jaw muscle coupling, vertical speed, and vertical displacement, and decreased lateral excursions of the mandible. Little is known about the impact of molar emergence on chewing motor development, although it is likely to be highly significant. The deciduous molars erupt from 13 to 33 months and the canines from 16 to 22 months. Molars are critical for generating the shearing forces that break down the bolus and for providing a consistent point of occlusal contact. The anterior motion of the jaw motion is constrained anteriorly by the incisors

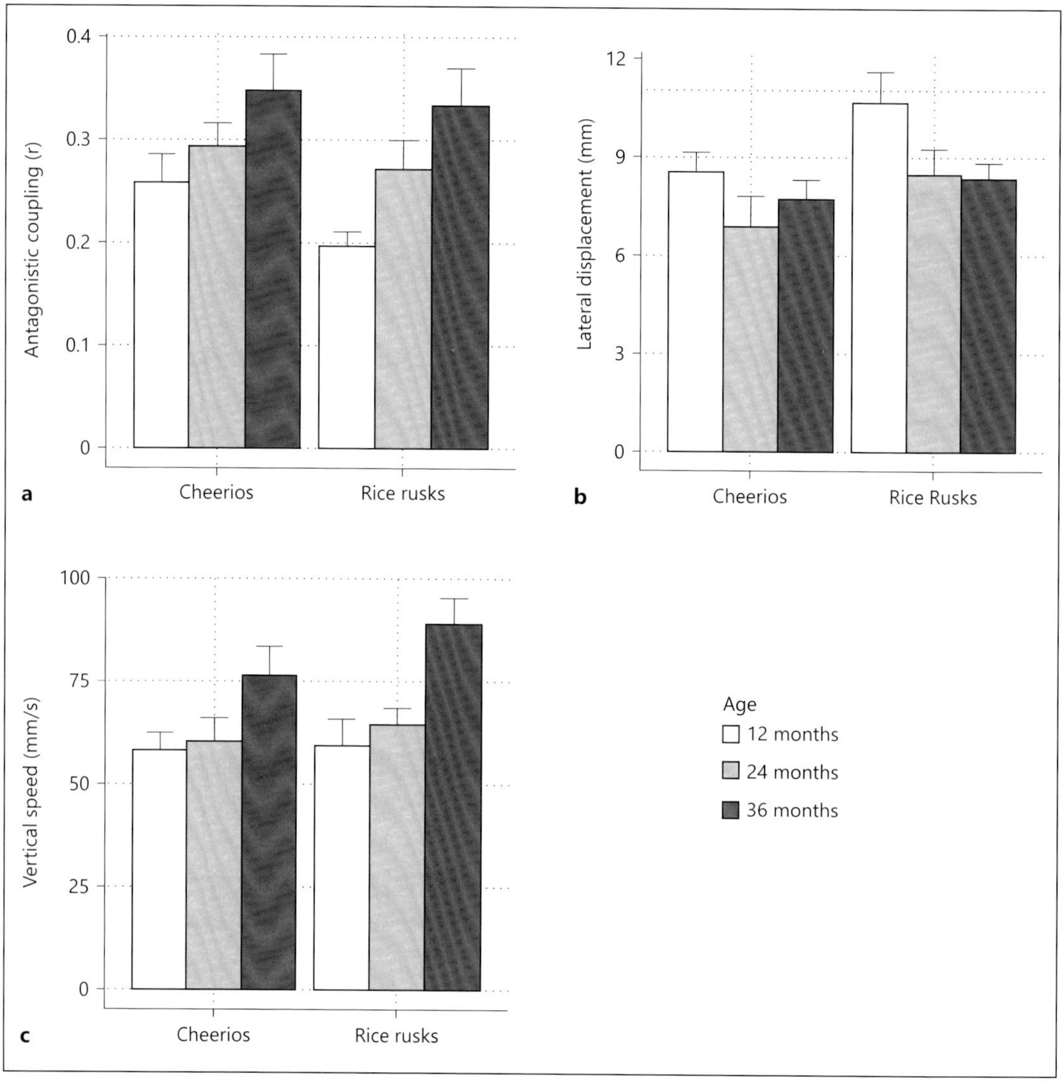

Fig. 3. With age, the jaw elevators and depressors became more tightly coupled (**a**). The beginning chewers (i.e. 12-month-olds) showed more lateral displacement than the advanced chewers (i.e. 24- and 36-month-olds) (**b**). Vertical speed of the jaw increased with age (**c**). For all three parameters, the greater age-related differences were for the Rice Rusks than the Cheerios.

and the cuspal anatomy of the molars, and posteriorly by the temporal mandibular joint. Therefore, prior to the eruption of molars, jaw movements during the occlusal phase of the chewing cycle (fig. 1) are likely to be less stable [10].

Although these findings are preliminary (i.e., only based on the testing of a small number of textures in a relatively small cohort of participants), our findings suggest that (1) the development of chewing solids is a protracted process extending well past the third year of life and (2) chewing motor development is characterized by two broad phases: a beginning and a refinement phase that appeared to be delineated by the emergence of molars, and (3) products with different textures can impact chewing abilities and learning how to chew.

In conclusion, chewing development and the factors that affect it, such as food texture, experience, and tooth emergence, are critical components to feeding readiness that have been largely ignored despite its importance for safe and successful early feeding experiences. Studying chewing motor development using biomechanical-based approaches will provide a more comprehensive understanding of the oromotor control and coordination required to safely and efficiently learn to chew.

Disclosure Statement

This research was sponsored by Nestec Ltd. and may lead to the development of products.

References

1 World Health Organization: Infant and Young Child Feeding: Model Chapter for Textbooks for Medical Students and Allied Health Professionals. Geneva, World Health Organization, 2009, http://whqlibdoc.who.int/publications/2009/9789241597494_eng.pdf.

2 Butte N, Cobb K, Dwyer J, et al: The start healthy feeding guidelines for infants and toddlers. J Am Diet Assoc 2004;104:442–454.

3 Clayton HB, Li R, Perrine CG, et al: Prevalence and reasons for introducing infants early to solid foods: variations by milk feeding type. Pediatrics 2013;131:e1108–3114.

4 Bril B, Hombessa-Nkounkou E, Bouville JF, et al: From milk to adult diet: a comparative study on the socialization of food. Food Foodways 2001;9:155–186.

5 Bright Futures: Nutrition Supervision. https://brightfutures.aap.org/Bright Futures Documents/BFNutrition3rdEditionSupervision.pdf (accessed August 4, 2016).

6 Committee on Injury, Violence and Poison Prevention: Prevention of choking among children. Pediatrics 2010;125:601–607.

7 Ahlgren J: Mechanism of mastication: a quantitative cinematographic and electromyographic study of mastication movements in children, with special reference to occlusion of the teeth. Acta Odontol Scand 1966; 24:5–109.

8 Green JR, Moore CA, Ruark JL, et al: Development of chewing in children from 12 to 48 months: longitudinal study of EMG patterns. J Neurophysiol 1997;77:2704–2716.

9 Steeve RW: Babbling and chewing: jaw kinematics from 8 to 22 months. J Phon 2010;38: 445–458.

10 Wilson EM, Green JR: The development of jaw motion for mastication. Early Hum Dev 2009;85:303–311.

11 Le Révérend BJD, Edelson LR, Loret C: Anatomical, functional, physiological and behavioural aspects of the development of mastication in early childhood. Br J Nutr 2014;111: 403–414.

12 Suzuki H, Fukushima M, Okamoto S, et al: Effects of thorough mastication on postprandial plasma glucose concentrations in nonobese Japanese subjects. Metabolism 2005;54: 1593–1599.

13 Hiiemae KM, Palmer JB: Food transport and bolus formation during complete feeding sequences on foods of different initial consistency. Dysphagia 1999;14:31–42.
14 Abed GS, Buschang PH, Taylor R, et al: Maturational and functional related differences in rat craniofacial growth. Arch Oral Biol 2007;52:1018–1025.
15 Luca L, Roberto D, Francesca SM, et al: Consistency of diet and its effects on mandibular morphogenesis in the young rat. Prog Orthod 2003;4:3–7.
16 Kiliaridis S, Shyu BC: Isometric muscle tension generated by masseter stimulation after prolonged alteration of the consistency of the diet fed to growing rats. Arch Oral Biol 1988; 33:467–472.
17 Corruccini R, Beecher R: Occlusal variation related to soft diet in a nonhuman primate. Science 1982;218:74–76.
18 Fujishita A, Koga Y, Utsumi D, et al: Effects of feeding a soft diet and subsequent rehabilitation on the development of the masticatory function. J Oral Rehabil 2015;42:266–274.
19 Harris G: Developmental, regulatory and cognitive aspects of feeding disorders; in Southall A, Schwartz A (eds): Feeding Problems in Children. Oxford, Radcliffe, 2000, pp 77–88.
20 Illingworth RS, Lister J: The critical or sensitive period, with special reference to certain feeding problems in infants and children. J Pediatr 1964;65:839–848.
21 Mason SJ, Harris G, Blissett J: Tube feeding in infancy: implications for the development of normal eating and drinking skills. Dysphagia 2005;20:46–61.
22 Nicklaus S: Children's acceptance of new foods at weaning. Role of practices of weaning and of food sensory properties. Appetite 2011;57:812–815.
23 Coulthard H, Harris G, Emmett P: Delayed introduction of lumpy foods to children during the complementary feeding period affects child's food acceptance and feeding at 7 years of age. Matern Child Nutr 2009;5:75–85.
24 Northstone K, Emmett P, Nethersole F: The effect of age of introduction to lumpy solids on foods eaten and reported feeding difficulties at 6 and 15 months. J Hum Nutr Diet 2001;14:43–54.
25 Blum-Kemelor DM (ed): Feeding Infants: A Guide for Use in the Child Nutrition Programs. Washington, United States Department of Agriculture, 2016, pp 43–59, http://www.fns.usda.gov/sites/default/files/feedinginfants-ch7.pdf.
26 Lund JP: Mastication and its control by the brain stem. Crit Rev Oral Biol Med 1991;2: 33–64.
27 Nakamura Y, Katakura N: Generation of masticatory rhythm in the brainstem. Neurosci Res 1995;23:1–19.
28 Mioche L, Peyron MA: Bite force displayed during assessment of hardness in various texture contexts. Arch Oral Biol 1995;40:415–423.
29 Grigoriadis A, Johansson RS, Trulsson M: Temporal profile and amplitude of human masseter muscle activity is adapted to food properties during individual chewing cycles. J Oral Rehabil 2014;41:367–373.
30 Gisel EG: Effect of food texture on the development of chewing of children between six months and two years of age. Dev Med Child Neurol 1991;33:69–79.

Black RE, Makrides M, Ong KK (eds): Complementary Feeding: Building the Foundations for a Healthy Life. Nestlé Nutr Inst Workshop Ser, vol 87, pp 39–48, (DOI: 10.1159/000448936)
Nestec Ltd., Vevey/S. Karger AG., Basel, © 2017

Update on Timing and Source of 'Allergenic' Foods

Debra J. Palmer

School of Paediatrics and Child Health, University of Western Australia, Princess Margaret Hospital, Subiaco, WA, Australia

Abstract

As the prevalence of food allergies in many communities continues to rise, the question of when in infancy to introduce any solid foods, or specific 'more allergenic' foods, as a food allergy prevention strategy has been debated. Observational studies have found that introducing any solid foods prior to 4 months of age was associated with an increased risk of allergic disease. Hence, the current allergy prevention consensus recommendation is that the introduction of any solid foods should commence after 4 months of age. Over recent years, several randomized controlled trials have been conducted to investigate the 'ideal' timing of introduction of some specific 'more allergenic' foods (including peanuts and eggs) into infant diets. To date, the results from three of these trials have determined that there is no reason to delay the introduction of the 'more allergenic' foods into the infant's diet after solid foods have commenced. However, these trials have also highlighted the finding that some infants are sensitized to food allergens before any known ingestion of solid foods. Thus, future research needs to focus on strategies to prevent early-life food allergen sensitization prior to complementary feeding.

Introduction

Over the past two decades, there has been considerable debate with regard to when and which foods should be introduced into the infants' diet, especially as an allergy prevention strategy. The need for high-quality evidence in this field of research remains a priority given; in many regions around the world, early-life food allergies appear to be increasing. In Australia, more than 10% of 1-year-olds have been found to have a challenge-proven food allergy [1], and the incidence of food-related anaphylaxis, most commonly experienced by preschool aged children, has also been identified to have increased further over the past decade [2]. Furthermore, this burden of food allergy in the community appears to be growing with the finding of increasing persistence of some food allergies into late childhood [3]. Hence, with increasing incidence, severity and persistence, effective food allergy prevention strategies are needed. Over the past few years, the quality of available evidence on this topic has begun to improve with the conduct of several randomized controlled trials (RCTs) investigating the effect of the timing of introduction of some solid foods on food allergy outcomes.

When to Introduce Any Solid Foods?

Observational studies have previously looked for associations of age at commencement of any solid foods with allergic disease outcomes, and either found no associations or that the introduction at less than 4 months of age was associated with increased risk of food allergy [4, 5]. The recently published Enquiring About Tolerance (EAT) Trial in the UK was an RCT which aimed to compare the commencement of solid foods in exclusively breastfed infants from 3 months of age to solid food avoidance with continued exclusive breastfeeding until around 6 months of age [6]. No differences in food allergy outcomes were found in this EAT trial [6], where 7.1% (42/595) of the infants in the group avoiding solid foods until 6 months developed food allergy compared to 5.6% (32/567) of the infants in the group with early introduction of solids from 3 months (relative risk 0.80; 95% CI 0.51–1.25; $p = 0.32$). Thus, the EAT Trial results do not support the need to change the existing current consensus in allergy prevention guidelines [7] that recommend the introduction of any solid foods into infant diets should commence after 4 months of age.

When to Introduce Specific 'More Allergenic' Foods?

In the year 2000, the American Academy of Pediatrics Committee on Nutrition recommended that for infants at higher risk of allergy (based on family history) that parents and carers should delay the introduction of 'more allergenic' foods in their diet. This recommendation included that cow's milk products be avoided until 1 year, eggs until 2 years, and nuts and fish until 3 years of age. Over the next few years, this delayed introduction to certain 'more allergenic' foods then became progressively incorporated into infant feeding guidelines in many countries. Then, in contrast, over the next decade, observational studies found that delayed introduction, beyond 6–10 months of age, of some specific foods (in-

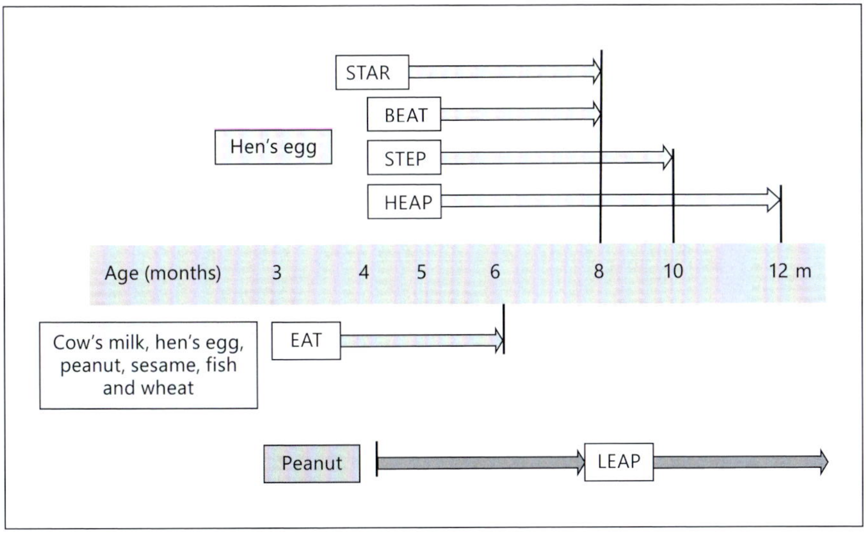

Fig. 1. Timing of and which specific food allergens were introduced during infancy in the intervention groups of the EAT, LEAP, BEAT, HEAP, STAR, and STEP RCTs.

cluding oats, wheat, dairy foods, fish, and egg) to be associated with increased risk of allergic disease, in particular eczema [8–13] and allergic sensitization [11, 12, 14–16]. With regard to specific food allergy outcomes, one cohort study [17] found that delayed egg introduction beyond 10 months was associated with a higher risk of egg allergy compared with earlier introduction at 4–6 months of age. In light of this observational evidence, there was then a major change in expert committee recommendations which now advise that for allergy prevention there is no benefit of delaying the introduction of 'more allergenic' foods in the diet of infants [7].

With the recognition that the level of evidence from these observational cohort studies was generally weak, at least six RCTs have been conducted in recent years to investigate whether the timing of introduction of specific food allergens into the infant diet reduces the risk of developing food allergy. Figure 1 summarizes the timing of and which specific foods were investigated in these RCTs: EAT, Learning Early About Peanut Allergy (LEAP), Beating Egg Allergy Trial (BEAT), Hen's Egg Allergy Prevention (HEAP), Solids Timing for Allergy Reduction (STAR), and Starting Time of Egg Protein (STEP) Trials. It is important to note some of the differences in trial design even between the five trials which investigated the timing of egg introduction. Some of these specific trial characteristics are summarized in table 1. The 'levels of risk' of potential food allergy development in the population of infants studied also need to be distinguished between several of the trials. This will potentially be an important distinguishing point between the var-

Table 1. RCTs including egg introduction in infancy to prevent egg allergy

Trial name (location)	Level of allergy risk and sample size	All egg-sensitized infants included	Blinded trial	Intervention period	Frequency and egg type
BEAT Trial (Australia)	Intermediate risk; family history of allergic disease(n = 319)	No	Yes	From 4–6 months of age until 8 months	Daily: whole pasteurized raw egg powder
EAT Trial (UK)	Normal risk; general population (n = 1,303)	No	No	From 3 months of age until 6 months	2 times per week: cooked (boiled) egg
HEAP Trial (Germany)	Normal risk; general population (n = 406)	No	Yes	From 4–6 Months of age	3 times per week: egg powder
STAR Trial (Australia)	High risk; moderate-to-severe eczema in infants (n = 86)	Yes	Yes	From 4 months of age until 8 months	Daily: whole pasteurized raw egg powder
STEP Trial (Australia)	Intermediate risk; atopic mothers but eczema absent in infants (n = 820)	Yes	Yes	From 4–6.5 months of age until 10 months	Daily: whole pasteurized raw egg powder

ious trial results and is an essential point to consider if, in the future, the results are to be translated into infant feeding allergy prevention guidelines.

Another critical difference between some of these trials involves the prescreening and exclusion of potential infant participants for sensitization to the food allergen(s) prior to randomization in the trial. In order to apply the results in practice from the LEAP, EAT, BEAT, and HEAP RCTs, infants will need to undergo skin prick testing or have food allergen-specific IgE blood testing prior to the introduction of the 'more allergenic' solid foods in their diets(s). This is neither practical nor feasible from a cost perspective in many communities. Hence, only the results from two of the egg intervention RCTs, the STAR Trial involving infants with moderate-to-severe eczema and the STEP Trial for infants without any eczema, can truly be translated and applied in the community setting without the need for testing infants prior to solid introduction of the 'more allergenic' foods.

Elements of the quality of trial design, for example blinding of participants, also need to be noted. The influence of reverse causation can only truly be eliminated with a prospective double-blind RCT design. Without blinded randomizations, as was the case in two of these recently published trials [6, 18], it is also more difficult to allow for other potential confounding factors. Although all of these six RCTs have now completed the participant intervention phases, to date the results from only three RCTs [6, 18, 19] have been published and will be discussed here. The results of the other three RCTs of egg introduction timing are anticipated within the next year, and the availability of these results will add greater clarity and contribute additional dimensions to the composite picture of available evidence to this area of food allergy prevention research.

The first of these RCTs to be published was the *STAR Trial,* which investigated the early regular inclusion of *eggs* in solid-food diets of infants at 'high risk' of developing egg allergy due to moderate-to-severe eczema prior to 4 months of age [19]. In this double-blind trial, the intervention group of infants was exposed to whole pasteurized raw egg powder mixed into their solid foods each day from 4 to 8 months of age, whereas the control group had rice powder. In the STAR Trial, 33% (14/42) of infants introduced to egg from 4 months of age developed an egg allergy at 12 months of age versus 51% (18/35) in the control group (relative risk 0.65; 95% CI 0.38–1.11; $p = 0.11$). Unfortunately, the results of this trial did not reach statistical significance due to the small sample size of the trial ($n = 86$). In the STAR Trial, 31% (15/49) of infants randomized to receive pasteurized raw egg powder had an allergic reaction to eggs at 4 months of age and did not continue the egg powder ingestion. This included 1 infant who had anaphylaxis at 4 months of age on the first ingestion of this egg powder. It has been proposed that this may have been due to the 'more allergenic' nature of pasteurized raw egg. However, it is worthy of mention here that 6 infants in the rice powder group of the STAR Trial [19] also had allergic reactions to the supervised first ingestion of cooked egg at 8 months of age, including 1 infant who had anaphylaxis upon the first ingestion of cooked (hard-boiled) egg. Thus reactions to both pasteurized raw and cooked egg occurred in a population of infants with moderate-to-severe eczema upon egg ingestion prior to 9 months of age. The recently completed STEP Trial will provide valuable insight into any possible differences in clinical allergic reaction rates to the introduction of egg in a population of infants with hereditary risk of allergic disease but without symptoms of eczema prior to randomization.

The results have also been published from the *LEAP Study,* which investigated the introduction and regular dietary intake of *peanuts,* commencing between 4 and 11 months of age, in the diet of infants compared to the avoidance of peanut in the child's diet until 5 years of age [18]. It is important to note that 9% (76/834) of the infants initially screened were found to have peanut sensitization (skin prick test: >4 mm) before any known peanut ingestion and were then subsequently excluded prior to randomization and recommended to continue to avoid peanut and peanut-containing products. Hence, both the safety and the effect of the introduction of peanuts during infancy for previously peanut-sensitized infants remains unknown. The results of this RCT, with excellent follow-up rates of 98%, found that the introduction of peanuts prior to 11 months of age, compared to avoidance until 5 years of age, did significantly reduce the incidence of peanut allergy at 5 years of age [18]. When translating the results from this LEAP RCT it is critical to note that there was a wide infant age range at randomization of 4–11 months, the average age of commencement of peanut introduction was around 8 months of age, and some infants did not start peanut ingestion until almost 11 months of age.

While most of these recent RCTs are targeting the effects of early feeding with one specific food, the *EAT Trial* was unique in investigating the sequential introduction of *cow's milk protein (yoghurt), cooked hen's egg, peanut, white fish, sesame, and wheat from 3 months,* compared to exclusive breastfeeding until around 6 months of age [6]. Although the target infant population for this study was the general population, it should be recognized that after recruitment more than 80% of the participating infants had a hereditary risk of allergy (with at least one parent with a history of allergic disease). This is higher than the 50–60% previously noted for the general infant population in the UK. As previously discussed, no differences in food allergy outcomes were found between the groups in the intention-to-treat results from this EAT trial [6]. Although the per-protocol results may appear to have shown a beneficial effect of the intervention with a food allergy rate of 2.4% (5/208) in the intervention group compared to 7.3% (38/524) in the control group (relative risk 0.33; 95% CI 0.13–0.83; $p = 0.01$), this result should be interpreted with caution as only 32% in the intervention group adhered to the trial protocol and had the primary outcome measured compared to 80% in the control group. One interesting finding from the EAT trial was that the consumption of 2 g of peanut or egg white protein per week was associated with a significantly lower prevalence of these respective food allergies than was associated with less consumption. Hence, this raises the concept that the induction of tolerance to food allergens in infancy may be dose dependent.

The rationale for the introduction of these food allergens in infancy RCTs is also based on animal studies, which demonstrated that the development of tolerance is an allergen-driven process through early regular oral exposure to food proteins. Both the STAR [19] and LEAP [18] Trials demonstrated that the food allergen (egg or peanut, respectively)-specific IgG4 levels were higher in the food allergen consumption group than in the avoidance group. This increase in specific IgG4 levels after regular ingestion of food allergens is consistent with findings from specific oral tolerance induction studies in food-allergic children [20]. Of particular interest in the LEAP Trial was the finding that elevated IgG4 levels were associated with the absence of an allergic reaction to peanut unless the child also had very high peanut-specific IgE levels. Hence, higher IgG4 levels appear to be associated with a protective role against the development of food allergy and appear responsive to modulation by early regular food allergen exposure.

Early-Infancy Food Allergen Sensitization prior to Solid Food Introduction

In the EAT, LEAP, and STAR RCTs [6, 18, 19, 21, 22], sensitization to food allergens was detected prior to the introduction of these specific foods into the infant's solid-food diet. Approximately one quarter of the infants in both the STAR and LEAP RCTs [18, 19, 21] had peanut sensitization (peanut-specific IgE levels ≥0.35 kU/l) and more than one third (35.8%) of the STAR Trial infants [19] had egg sensitization (egg-specific IgE levels ≥0.35 kU/l) at baseline prior to the introduction of these food allergens in their solid foods. Although not all infants who are sensitized to a food allergen will have an allergic reaction upon ingestion to that food, in the STAR Trial the majority of these egg-sensitized infants had a clinical allergic reaction upon the first known oral exposure to egg-containing foods [19]. Analysis of the early T-cell responses to egg proteins in the STAR Trial infants determined that those 4-month-old infants who subsequently developed egg allergy already had significantly higher Th2 cytokine responses to multiple egg protein allergens, particularly elevated IL-13 responses to ovalbumin ($p = 0.004$), ovomucoid ($p = 0.012$), and lysozyme ($p = 0.003$), and elevated IL-5 to the same antigens ($p = 0.031$, 0.04 and 0.003, respectively) [23]. IL-13 responses to ovalbumin and lysozyme, and IL-5 responses to lysozyme at 4 months significantly predicted egg allergy at 12 months, and this did not appear to be modified by 'early' introduction of egg into solid foods [23]. Thus, a 'critical time' to investigate intervention strategies to reduce food allergy development appears to be early in life prior to complementary feeding.

Sensitization in early infancy where there was no previous history of known direct ingestion of the specific food allergens in solid foods by the infant [6, 18, 19, 22] indicates previous exposure through other routes potentially through the cutaneous barrier, breast milk or in utero. The initial route of food allergen exposure may be an important determinant of either the development of sensitization or oral tolerance during infancy. Early oral exposure to allergens through the gut is critical for maintaining and reinforcing oral tolerance, and food allergens secreted in breast milk may be an important potential early source. In animal studies, allergen exposure through maternal milk has been shown to induce oral tolerance [24]. Although common food allergen proteins have been detected in human breast milk, including peanut [24, 25] and egg protein [26, 27], their role in the development of oral tolerance in human breastfed infants remains unknown.

Without oral food allergen exposure, there is concern that exposure through the skin is more likely to induce sensitization, particularly in children with impaired cutaneous barrier function, including infants with eczema [28]. This is thought to occur when infants are exposed to low levels of food allergens at potentially sensitizing doses in their environment [29]. Food allergens have been detected in house dust and in the bedding of young children [30]. Household consumption of peanut has been found to be positively correlated with peanut levels detected in house dust samples [30] and have also been associated with increased risk of peanut allergy [29]. It has been proposed that early-life cutaneous exposure in the absence of oral exposure leads to allergic sensitization, whereas high levels of oral exposure lead to tolerance irrespective of environmental exposure [28]. Further research is still needed to address the continued uncertainty with regard to the role and mechanisms of early food allergen encounter, and how variations in the context of food allergen exposure can influence the risk of sensitization.

Conclusions

The current allergy prevention consensus recommendation is that the introduction of solid foods should commence after 4 months of age. Recent RCT evidence indicates that there appears to be no reason to delay the introduction of the 'more allergenic' foods (including egg and peanut) into the infant's diet after the ingestion of solid foods has commenced. Prevention of food allergen sensitization in early infancy, prior to the commencement of solid foods, should be a focus of future research as a food allergy prevention strategy.

Disclosure Statement

The author has no conflicts of interest to declare in relation to this publication.

References

1 Osborne NJ, Koplin JJ, Martin PE, et al: Prevalence of challenge-proven IgE-mediated food allergy using population-based sampling and predetermined challenge criteria in infants. J Allergy Clin Immunol 2011;127:668–676.e1-2.
2 Mullins RJ, Dear KB, Tang ML: Time trends in Australian hospital anaphylaxis admissions in 1998–1999 to 2011–2012. J Allergy Clin Immunol 2015;136:367–375.
3 Savage JH, Matsui EC, Skripak JM, Wood RA: The natural history of egg allergy. J Allergy Clin Immunol 2007;120:1413–1417.

4 Grimshaw KE, Maskell J, Oliver EM, et al: Introduction of complementary foods and the relationship to food allergy. Pediatrics 2013;132:e1529–e1538.
5 Kajosaari M, Saarinen UM: Prophylaxis of atopic disease by six months' total solid food elimination. Evaluation of 135 exclusively breast-fed infants of atopic families. Acta Paediatr Scand 1983;72:411–414.
6 Perkin MR, Logan K, Tseng A, et al: Randomized trial of introduction of allergenic foods in breast-fed infants. N Engl J Med 2016;374:1733–1743.
7 Muraro A, Halken S, Arshad SH, et al: EAACI food allergy and anaphylaxis guidelines. Primary prevention of food allergy. Allergy 2014;69:590–601.
8 Alm B, Aberg N, Erdes L, et al: Early introduction of fish decreases the risk of eczema in infants. Arch Dis Child 2009;94:11–15.
9 Filipiak B, Zutavern A, Koletzko S, et al: Solid food introduction in relation to eczema: results from a four-year prospective birth cohort study. J Pediatr 2007;151:352–358.
10 Hesselmar B, Saalman R, Rudin A, et al: Early fish introduction is associated with less eczema, but not sensitization, in infants. Acta Paediatr 2010;99:1861–1867.
11 Kull I, Bergstrom A, Lilja G, et al: Fish consumption during the first year of life and development of allergic diseases during childhood. Allergy 2006;61:1009–1015.
12 Snijders BE, Thijs C, van Ree R, van den Brandt PA: Age at first introduction of cow milk products and other food products in relation to infant atopic manifestations in the first 2 years of life: the KOALA Birth Cohort Study. Pediatrics 2008;122:e115–e122.
13 Zutavern A, von Mutius E, Harris J, et al: The introduction of solids in relation to asthma and eczema. Arch Dis Child 2004;89:303–308.
14 Nwaru BI, Erkkola M, Ahonen S, et al: Age at the introduction of solid foods during the first year and allergic sensitization at age 5 years. Pediatrics 2010;125:50–59.
15 Nwaru BI, Takkinen HM, Niemela O, et al: Introduction of complementary foods in infancy and atopic sensitization at the age of 5 years: timing and food diversity in a Finnish birth cohort. Allergy 2013;68:507–516.
16 Zutavern A, Brockow I, Schaaf B, et al: Timing of solid food introduction in relation to eczema, asthma, allergic rhinitis, and food and inhalant sensitization at the age of 6 years: results from the prospective birth cohort study LISA. Pediatrics 2008;121:e44–e52.
17 Koplin JJ, Osborne NJ, Wake M, et al: Can early introduction of egg prevent egg allergy in infants? A population-based study. J Allergy Clin Immunol 2010;126:807–813.
18 Du Toit G, Roberts G, Sayre PH, et al: Randomized trial of peanut consumption in infants at risk for peanut allergy. N Engl J Med 2015;372:803–813.
19 Palmer DJ, Metcalfe J, Makrides M, et al: Early regular egg exposure in infants with eczema: a randomized controlled trial. J Allergy Clin Immunol 2013;132:387–392.e1.
20 Burks AW, Jones SM, Wood RA, et al: Oral immunotherapy for treatment of egg allergy in children. N Engl J Med 2012;367:233–243.
21 Du Toit G, Roberts G, Sayre PH, et al: Identifying infants at high risk of peanut allergy: the Learning Early About Peanut Allergy (LEAP) screening study. J Allergy Clin Immunol 2013;131:135–143.e1-12.
22 Perkin MR, Logan K, Marrs T, et al: Enquiring About Tolerance (EAT) study: feasibility of an early allergenic food introduction regimen. J Allergy Clin Immunol 2016;137:1477–1486.e8.
23 Metcalfe JR, D'Vaz N, Makrides M, et al: Elevated IL-5 and IL-13 responses to egg proteins predate the introduction of egg in solid foods in infants with eczema. Clin Exp Allergy 2016;46:308–316.
24 Bernard H, Ah-Leung S, Drumare MF, et al: Peanut allergens are rapidly transferred in human breast milk and can prevent sensitization in mice. Allergy 2014;69:888–897.
25 Vadas P, Wai Y, Burks W, Perelman B: Detection of peanut allergens in breast milk of lactating women. JAMA 2001;285:1746–1748.
26 Palmer DJ, Gold MS, Makrides M: Effect of cooked and raw egg consumption on ovalbumin content of human milk: a randomized, double-blind, cross-over trial. Clin Exp Allergy 2005;35:173–178.

27 Vance GH, Lewis SA, Grimshaw KE, et al: Exposure of the fetus and infant to hens' egg ovalbumin via the placenta and breast milk in relation to maternal intake of dietary egg. Clin Exp Allergy 2005;35:1318–1326.
28 Lack G: Epidemiologic risks for food allergy. J Allergy Clin Immunol 2008;121:1331–1336.
29 Fox AT, Sasieni P, du Toit G, et al: Household peanut consumption as a risk factor for the development of peanut allergy. J Allergy Clin Immunol 2009;123:417–423.
30 Brough HA, Santos AF, Makinson K, et al: Peanut protein in household dust is related to household peanut consumption and is biologically active. J Allergy Clin Immunol 2013;132:630–638.

Update on Introduction of Complementary Feeding

Black RE, Makrides M, Ong KK (eds): Complementary Feeding: Building the Foundations for a Healthy Life. Nestlé Nutr Inst Workshop Ser, vol 87, pp 49–58, (DOI: 10.1159/000448937)
Nestec Ltd., Vevey/S. Karger AG., Basel, © 2017

Flavor and Taste Development in the First Years of Life

Erin Sundseth Ross

Feeding Fundamentals, LLC., Thornton, CO, and University of Colorado, School of Medicine, Department of Pediatrics, Center for Family and Infant Interaction USA, Denver, CO, USA

Abstract

Across the first four years of life, infants transition from a diet of liquids to solid foods. Flavor preferences affect the acceptance of novel foods. Fetuses experience flavors in the uterine environment, and some preferences appear to be innate. Sweet and salty foods tend to be accepted by most newborns, while bitter tastes are rejected. Breast fed infants appear to have an advantage over formula fed infants, as their exposure to a varying flavor profile is influenced by the mother's diet. Infants are fairly accepting of novel foods, but rejection of new foods increases across the initial years of life. Children learn to accept novel foods through a variety of experiences, provided within social contexts. Some children are more accepting of various sensory inputs present during mealtimes. Parents report a greater challenge getting multiple taste exposures when their child exhibits less sensory adaptability. The number of foods eaten as a young child has a strong influence on the food repertoire later in childhood. Foods eaten by parents significantly predict the number and types of foods eaten by children. Strategies to help parents be more successful in achieving taste exposures in a positive social environment need to be identified.

Introduction

Data suggest that children with greater experiences with either flavors or textures during the complementary feeding period are more accepting of complex textures and eat a more varied diet [1, 2]. Early food experiences include direct experiences with flavors, smells and textures, as well as indirect experiences through exposures provided by caregivers. Direct experiences begin in utero, as the fetus tastes flavors transmitted through the amniotic fluid. Basic flavor preferences for sweet and salty flavors, and a dislike for bitter flavors, are apparent even in both the fetal and neonatal periods. However, these basic preferences are modifiable through a variety of direct and indirect experiences as the infant and young child transitions from liquid to puree and finally to textured foods. Parents play a significant role in providing a variety of exposures during the complementary feeding period.

Recent reviews of the fetus' and newborn's acceptance of the basic flavors bitter, salty, and sweet show infants appear to accept sweet flavors immediately while rejecting flavors with a bitter profile [3, 4]. Salty flavor also appears to be preferred over bitter, and a preference for salt appears to be reinforced by experiences [5]. Preliminary data indicate a preference for increased liking of salty tastes at 6 months increases liking for taste of salt at preschool ages as well [6]. There does not appear to be a correlation between intake of salty tastes at birth and preference at 2 years of age; a preference at 6 months is correlated to that at 2 years [6]. This may be due to the infant's changing preferences correlated with repeated exposures. Adding salt to novel vegetables appears to increase the acceptance of that food, supporting the hypothesis that salt is probably an innate preference [7].

Flavors across the First Years

Neonatal Period

The newborn infant's awareness of and discrimination for smells and flavors is well developed. Preliminary data suggest there may be flavors or smells that are naturally preferred by infants. Within hours of birth, infants with no prior experience with tastes other than those experienced within the uterine environment differentiate sour, bitter, sweet, and non-sweet taste stimuli, although all of the stimuli with the exception of sweet result in negative facial expressions through the brows and midface [3]. The amount of fluid the infant eats does not appear to be related to their facial expression of liking. Infants continue to prefer (like) and eat (ingest) more sweetened flavors over other flavors through the first 6 months of life.

Breastfed infants are exposed to varying flavors in their mother's milk and respond to flavor changes in the milk with changes in sucking patterns. Mennella [8] has focused on this exposure, and a recent review article summarizes this research. Data suggest breastfed infants are more accepting of a wider variety of foods in the weaning period, and the acceptance is not flavor specific [9, 10]. Mothers will typically provide similar foods to their infants during the complementary feeding period that they eat themselves. Increased acceptance is related to whether the mother's diet is rich in fruits and vegetables; eating these foods provides these flavors through the breastmilk. Exclusively breastfed children are more likely to consume more vegetables as preschoolers, but the threshold appears to be breastfeeding at least through 3 months of age [11]. This might be a reflection of early learning that occurs through the variety of flavors experienced during breastfeeding, given the diet of the mother. There does not appear to be a benefit of longer exclusive breastfeeding on vegetable consumption in young children [11].

Unlike breastfed infants, formula-fed infants do not experience a variety of flavors from feeding to feeding. Most parents give their child the same formula every feeding, every day, which limits their exposure to a variety of flavors. However, infants can demonstrate that they are learning from their taste experiences with formula as well. Data from a series of studies on acceptance and flavor learning associated with hydrolysate-containing formulas (HCF), which have more pronounced savory, bitter, and sour taste and stronger odors than cow's milk formula or human breast milk, suggest a preference develops that is brand specific [12]. This research has been summarized by Mennella and Ventura [13] in a review as well. There appears to be a sensitive period for accepting these flavors. Infants fed HCFs prior to 3.5 to 4 months of age readily accept it, and after eating a non-HCF will return to the HCF with less difficulty than those who were never fed HCFs. Infants reject HCFs when they are initially introduced to this formula after 4–5 months of age. By 4–5 years of age, children fed HCFs prefer similar flavor compounds in foods as are present in HCFs [14]. However, by 6–7 years of age, the influence of early exposure to HCFs appears to diminish and there is no correlation with a preference for sour or bitter flavors [14].

Weaning

With the introduction to solid foods, even pureed foods, texture must be considered as a sensory input along with taste [15]. Data suggest infants increase their acceptance of a food after repeated experience with that food, and increased exposure may generalize to novel foods [1, 16, 17]. However, it is unclear whether this generalized acceptance is for foods across nutrition categories or limited to other foods within that same category. Repeatedly giving the same food will increase acceptance of that food; giving a variety of fruits, meal to meal, appears to increase a general acceptance for fruits, but does not influence a similar generalized acceptance of vegetables. Changing variety of vegetables daily, or even during a meal (over repeatedly offering the same vegetable for a series of consecutive days), appears to increase consumption and liking of novel vegetables [17]. Within-meal variety (alternating 1–2 spoonfuls at a time of two or more foods) also appears to increase acceptance of the foods to which the infant is exposed, as well as to novel fruits and vegetables. Recent reviews summarize the current knowledge regarding the effect of repeated exposure on acceptance of flavors [15, 18]. During the beginning of the weaning period (typically at 5–7 months of age), a majority of foods are accepted and no clear rejection of the most bitter- or sour-tasting foods is evident [19]. However, not all children react the same to novel foods, and some will require more exposures to accept novel foods. The number of exposures necessary when introducing pureed foods is unclear, but it appears to be more than one or two, and generally not more than eight exposures [17]. A recent study by Caton et al. [20] suggests that intrinsic differences in sensory abilities may be interfering with accepting specific flavors, as some infants accept novel foods readily, whereas others do not appear to eat more even with repeated exposures.

Textured Foods

As children transition to textured foods, they must learn to accept a variety of both flavors and textures. Additionally, the physical skills required to eat these foods are much more complex. Food pickiness typically develops between the end of the first and second year [18]. Most children appear quite accepting of new foods within a few trials when introduced under the age of 1 year; food refusals increase significantly thereafter, and by 3 years of age children often reject foods previously accepted. One reason children begin to reject foods is likely that they acquire language and use language to exert control over their world. Saying 'no' is a powerful way to express their likes and dislikes. Fortunately, early exposure to a variety of foods may decrease the risk of becoming a picky eater. Children exposed to mashed foods prior to 9 months of age eat more fruits and vegetables at 7 years of age than those exposed after 9 months of age [11]. Introduction to home-cooked vegetables later than 6 months and decreased frequency of exposure are related to decreased consumption and variety at 7 years of age [21]. Commercially prepared pureed foods do not appear to have the same effect on increased consumption. This may be due to the consistent flavor/texture of commercially prepared foods compared to the slight variety provided when home-cooked fruits and vegetables are offered. Frequent exposure of home-cooked vegetables overcomes any correlation with consumption and variety at 7 years of age, even in the child introduced after 6 months of age [21]. Frequency of consumption of fruits, vegetables, and sweets at 1 year of age significantly predicts their consumption at 2 years of age [22].

Generally, a liking for vegetables appears to be learned, rather than innate [23, 24]. Without direction, preschool children frequently avoid choosing vegetables as part of a meal [25]. Having a child take a 'small taste' of a vegetable does increase liking for the target food, and allowing the child to spit out the food increases their willingness to try the food [23]. Taste exposure to novel foods is the most effective and long-lasting strategy for increasing acceptance of novel foods, and flavor-flavor learning strategies (pairing a novel food with a preferred flavor) have some support for them as well. Visual or olfactory exposure alone does not appear to influence acceptance. The effectiveness of flavor-flavor strategies is likely due to the increased taste exposure, as the child is more willing to try the novel food using this strategy [24].

What is clear is that a child's food preferences are solidifying early in life, and younger children are more malleable than older children [26]. Additionally, food-related variety in the first 2 years strongly influences dietary variety in school-aged children. Even though children are exposed to foods outside of the family home, by 8 years of age their preferences are still primarily formed by what their mother prefers [27]. This is in large part due to the fact that mothers rarely offer foods to their children that they themselves dislike [27]. Given that parental preferences are such a strong influencing factor on children's exposure to foods, it is important for parents to offer a wide variety of foods during the complementary feeding period. However, the average number of exposures to non-preferred foods, reported by parents, is two to three [27]. Parents often stop offering foods that are not readily accepted by their children.

Future Directions

With all of this understanding regarding flavor and taste development, research suggests that children are not benefitting from our increased knowledge. While research has clarified the role of the parent and described a number of strategies designed to improve the variety of foods in a child's repertoire, children's acceptance of age-appropriate, nutrient-dense foods has not improved. The prevalence of overweight and obesity in children has doubled in the last 30 years, and 25–30% of children in the US do not consume appropriate amounts of fruits and vegetables [28]. Research is focusing on the complex interaction between the child and the parent during mealtimes. In a study of children from three countries, Caton et al. [20] found that there were four 'categories' of child eating styles. Forty percent of infants 4–38 months of age were considered 'learners' and steadily increased in their consumption of a novel puree with repeated exposure; an additional 21% readily ate >75% of the novel puree at every exposure (i.e., did not need repeated exposures) and were categorized as 'plate cleaners'. Parents of 'learners and plate cleaners' are reinforced to offer a variety of foods because their child readily accepts these experiences. Sixteen percent of infants in this study were classified as 'noneaters', because they did not increase their consumption and in fact ate less than 10 g of the vegetable puree even at the fifth exposure. For parents of 'noneaters', offering a food repeatedly does not appear to be an effective strategy. These parents may 'give up' and stop offering novel foods, which may not be the appropriate response but is understandable. The remaining children (23%) did not appear to have a consistent pattern. Plate clearers enjoyed food more than noneaters, and noneaters scored highest on food fussiness [20]. The child's skills, abilities, innate characteristics, and experiential learning patterns are less understood than parental characteristics at this time, but clearly these child characteristics are influencing their acceptance of foods.

Fruits and vegetables have a bitter/sour flavor palate, which is the most challenging from a sensory standpoint. These foods also require the most sophisticated oral-motor movement pattern and correct placement in the mouth, making them more challenging. Liquids and purees require only a vertical movement of the mouth. Textured foods require that (1) the tongue moves laterally to place the food appropriately on the teeth, (2) the lateral edges of the tongue and the cheek keep the food in place, and (3) the jaw mashes the food. Some foods require a vertical chewing motion and quickly break apart and/or melt (e.g., soft cookies). Foods like raw vegetables require chewing patterns that are vertical, lateral, and diagonal (e.g., rotary chewing).

Both the parent and the child bring characteristics to the mealtime situation that influence their own actions and the other's actions. While research to date has focused primarily on the role of the parent, and described 'parenting styles', clearly a responsive parent may inadvertently resort to 'antistrategies' when their child is more difficult to feed. For instance, if a child refuses to eat a 'healthy diet' (perhaps because of minor skill issues), a parent who is worried about their child's weight gain may resort to letting their child eat only preferred foods. In fact, this alteration in the parent-child interaction during mealtimes has been identified in research focused on children with pediatric feeding disorders (skill-based disorders that influence a child's ability to eat a wide variety of foods to meet their growth and nutritional needs). Mothers of children with pediatric feeding disorders become more intrusive and less structured as their child's weight falters, and the more worried the mother is about her child's poor weight gain, the more her interactions during mealtime are affected [29]. While offering only preferred foods to the child is not an effective strategy for increasing food acceptance, the parent who does not understand the underlying reasons for refusal may lack the knowledge to provide alternative, more effective strategies.

Responsive feeding has been characterized as a parent being aware of an infant's cues (communication), assigning meaning to the cues, and responding

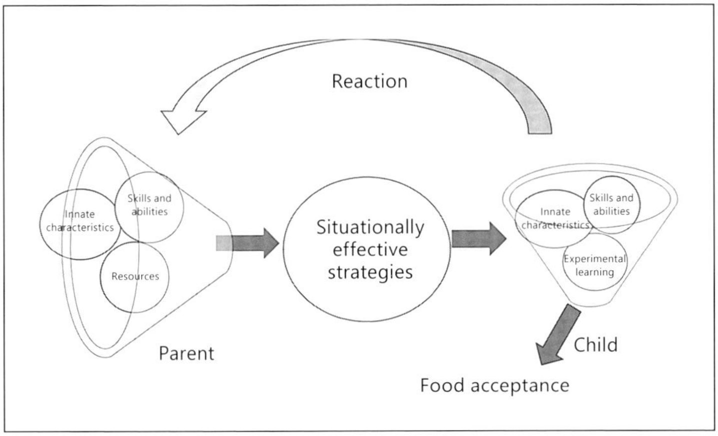

Fig. 1. Responsive feeding model for situationally effective strategies.

appropriately [30]. This has primarily been related to hunger and satiety cues. One might argue that a responsive parent, when interacting with a child who is not a plate cleaner or learner, might appropriately be trying alternative strategies in an attempt to support their child. In fact, in 2009, Farrow et al. [31] found parents may use different strategies within the same family, depending upon the child's needs. Eighty parents of two-sibling children reported using greater restrictive feeding practices with the fussier child than with the 'good eater'. They also reported using more pressure to eat with the siblings who were slower to eat, were fussier, under-ate, enjoyed food less, were less responsive to food, and were more responsive to internal satiety cues [31]. While this line of inquiry has been identified within the field of pediatric feeding disorders, it is likely that the parent of a 'picky eater' or even a child who is overweight or obese might be resorting to strategies that are not helpful as well.

Moving towards a More Responsive Feeding Model

In order to capitalize on the wealth of knowledge available from a nutrition standpoint regarding flavor and taste development, it is time to look at the effectiveness of strategies designed to improve the acceptance of novel foods in the context of a relationship. The child's behaviors influence the parent's behaviors, much like the parent influences the child. Figure 1 advances a new model for supporting food acceptance. In this model, the characteristics of both the parent and the child are considered. Table 1 describes characteristics of both the parent and the child that influence their interactions during mealtimes. Skills and

Table 1. Characteristics that influence the feeding environment

Skills and abilities	
Parent	
	Own likes/dislikes
	Knowledge regarding feeding strategies
	Ability to role model
	Awareness and responsiveness to a child's needs
	Ability to structure/manage mealtimes
	Knowledge of child development/nutrition
Child	
	Oromotor skills, gross/fine motor skills
	Sensory abilities
	Cognitive abilities/developmental age
Innate characteristics	
Parent	
	Temperament
	Beliefs
Child	
	Temperament
	Genetic taste capabilities
Resources of the parent	
Time	
Food availability	
Financial resources/socioeconomic factor	
Experiential learning of the child	
Familiarity of flavor	
Feedback from food (both positive and negative)	
Social context	
Reinforcement of behavior (both positive and negative)	

abilities as well as innate characteristics are categories that are shared. Resources of the family (e.g., the time available to prepare foods from scratch, financial resources to purchase foods, and available food options) and child experiences (e.g., previous experiences with the food) also influence the eventual acceptance of novel foods. A child is learning from every eating experience, and some of those experiences may be negative. For instance, a child may have food intolerances that are causing gastric distress; they may 'learn' that eating unknown, novel foods is an experience to be avoided.

The parent may offer foods that are appropriate, and the environment and basic strategies are appropriate. However, the child's response (influenced by their skills and abilities, innate characteristics, and experiential learning history) provides feedback to the parent. If the child's response is negative (e.g., gagging, crying, and throwing the food), the parent may not offer the food again. In this case, the strategies may end up becoming 'antistrategies'. By understanding how the child's characteristics influence the success of typical strategies, we can better educate the parent of the child who is a 'noneater', 'picky' or even a child who is overeating energy-dense but nutrient-lacking foods to use situationally appropriate strategies. The parent can then more effectively guide the mealtimes and provide effective strategies that support the child's food acceptance, while modifying their own behavior in response to the child's reactions during mealtimes. Rather than suggesting that the same strategies work for every child, the future direction for research focused on childhood nutrition needs to identify strategies that recognize the influence of both the parent and the child during mealtimes. This is a complex endeavor, but one that is a logical next step.

Disclosure Statement

The author declares that no financial or other conflict of interest exists in relation to the contents of the chapter.

References

1 Maier AS, Chabanet C, Schaal B, et al: Breastfeeding and experience with variety early in weaning increase infants' acceptance of new foods for up to two months. Clin Nutr 2008; 27:849–857.
2 Blossfeld I, Collins A, Kiely M, Delahunty C: Texture preferences of 12-month-old infants and the role of early experiences. Food Quality Preference 2007;18:396–404.
3 Rosenstein D, Oster H: Differential facial responses to four basic tastes in newborns. Child Dev 1988;59:1555–1568.
4 Mennella JA, Bobowski NK: The sweetness and bitterness of childhood: insights from basic research on taste preferences. Physiol Behav 2015;152:502–507.
5 Mennella JA, Reiter AR, Daniels LM: Vegetable and fruit acceptance during infancy: impact of ontogeny, genetics, and early experiences. Adv Nutr 2016;7:211S–219S.
6 Stein LJ, Cowart BJ, Beauchamp GK: The development of salty taste acceptance is related to dietary experience in human infants: a prospective study. Am J Clin Nutr 2012;95: 123–129.
7 Bouhlal S, Issanchou S, Chabanet C, Nicklaus S: 'Just a pinch of salt'. An experimental comparison of the effect of repeated exposure and flavor-flavor learning with salt or spice on vegetable acceptance in toddlers. Appetite 2014;83:209–217.
8 Mennella JA: Ontogeny of taste preferences: basic biology and implications for health. Am J Clin Nutr 2014;99:704S–711S.
9 Forestell CA, Mennella JA: Early determinants of fruit and vegetable acceptance. Pediatrics 2007;120:1247–1254.
10 Hausner H, Nicklaus S, Issanchou S, et al: Breastfeeding facilitates acceptance of a novel dietary flavour compound. Clin Nutr 2010; 29:141–148.
11 Coulthard H, Harris G, Emmett P: Delayed introduction of lumpy foods to children during the complementary feeding period affects child's food acceptance and feeding at 7 years of age. Matern Child Nutr 2009;5:75–85.
12 Mennella JA, Beauchamp GK: Understanding the origin of flavor preferences. Chem Senses 2005;30(suppl 1):i242–i243.

13 Mennella JA, Ventura AK: Early feeding: setting the stage for healthy eating habits, Nestle Nutrition workshop series. Nestle Nutr Workshop Ser Pediatr Program 2011;68:153–163; discussion 164–168.
14 Liem DG, Mennella JA: Sweet and sour preferences during childhood: role of early experiences. Dev Psychobiol 2002;41:388–395.
15 Johnson SL: Developmental and environmental influences on young children's vegetable preferences and consumption. Adv Nutr 2016;7:220S–231S.
16 Hausner H, Nicklaus S, Issanchou S, et al: Breastfeeding facilitates acceptance of a novel dietary flavour compound. Clin Nutr 2009; 29:141–148.
17 Mennella JA, Nicklaus S, Jagolino AL, Yourshaw LM: Variety is the spice of life: strategies for promoting fruit and vegetable acceptance during infancy. Physiol Behav 2008;94: 29–38.
18 Nicklaus S: The role of food experiences during early childhood in food pleasure learning. Appetite 2016;104:3–9.
19 Schwartz C, Chabanet C, Lange C, et al: The role of taste in food acceptance at the beginning of complementary feeding. Physiol Behav 2011;104:646–652.
20 Caton SJ, Blundell P, Ahern SM, et al: Learning to eat vegetables in early life: the role of timing, age and individual eating traits. PLoS One 2014;9:e97609.
21 Coulthard H, Harris G, Emmett P: Long-term consequences of early fruit and vegetable feeding practices in the United Kingdom. Public Health Nutr 2010;13:2044–2051.
22 Gregory JE, Paxton SJ, Brozovic AM: Maternal feeding practices predict fruit and vegetable consumption in young children. Results of a 12-month longitudinal study. Appetite 2011;57:167–172.
23 Anzman-Frasca S, Savage JS, Marini ME, et al: Repeated exposure and associative conditioning promote preschool children's liking of vegetables. Appetite 2012;58:543–553.
24 Hausner H, Olsen A, Moller P: Mere exposure and flavour-flavour learning increase 2–3 year-old children's acceptance of a novel vegetable. Appetite 2012;58:1152–1159.
25 Nicklaus S, Boggio V, Issanchou S: Food choices at lunch during the third year of life: high selection of animal and starchy foods but avoidance of vegetables. Acta Paediatr 2005;94:943–951.
26 Liem DG, Zandstra L, Thomas A: Prediction of children's flavour preferences. Effect of age and stability in reported preferences. Appetite 2010;55:69–75.
27 Skinner JD, Carruth BR, Wendy B, Ziegler PJ: Children's food preferences: a longitudinal analysis. J Am Diet Assoc 2002;102:1638–1647.
28 Fox MK, Condon E, Briefel RR, et al: Food consumption patterns of young preschoolers: are they starting off on the right path? J Am Diet Assoc 2010;110:S52–S59.
29 Gueron-Sela N, Atzaba-Poria N, Meiri G, Yerushalmi B: Maternal worries about child underweight mediate and moderate the relationship between child feeding disorders and mother-child feeding interactions. J Pediatr Psychol 2011;36:827–836.
30 Hodges EA, Hughes SO, Hopkinson J, Fisher JO: Maternal decisions about the initiation and termination of infant feeding. Appetite 2008;50:333–339.
31 Farrow CV, Galloway AT, Fraser K: Sibling eating behaviours and differential child feeding practices reported by parents. Appetite 2009;52:307–312.

Black RE, Makrides M, Ong KK (eds): Complementary Feeding: Building the Foundations for a Healthy Life. Nestlé Nutr Inst Workshop Ser, vol 87, pp 59–61, (DOI: 10.1159/000449498)

Summary of Update on Introduction of Complementary Feeding

The first session of the workshop focused on the importance of early life nutrition, and the important role early-life feeding plays in forming early food preferences and food behaviors that influence longer-term health.

The first speaker, *Merryn J. Netting* and *Maria Makrides* set the scene for the workshop by describing the changing nutritional requirements of 6- to 12-month-olds progressing into the second year of life. Energy and protein, iron, and zinc were identified as nutrients of risk in the second 6 months of life, and while iron, zinc, and iodine requirements remain similar, B-group vitamins and calcium needs increase in the second year of age with a relative per kilo drop in energy and protein requirements. The potential of delayed cord clamping after birth to improve iron status in the second 6 months of life was discussed. Complementary feeding guidelines vary from lower- to higher-income countries; however, despite the guidelines, dietary intake surveys have identified that low dietary variety amongst young children is a universal issue.

Jacqueline F. Gould reviewed evidence related to complementary feeding, micronutrients, and developmental outcomes of children. The first 2 years is a time of crucial brain development where high caloric intake is necessary to allow creation of new synapses, maintenance of established synapses, myelination, and every-day psychological functioning. Key nutrients needed for infant brain development include iron, fatty acids, and protein, and deficiencies in key nutrients during the early feeding period have been consistently linked to child development outcomes. However, due to methodological and study design issues, this is yet to be proven by randomized controlled trials. Given the significant development that takes place during this period on later health outcomes, national and international public health policies to improve infant nutrition may be an effective means of improving general population health. However, there is a need for future, large, quality randomized controlled trials investigating the role of specific nutrients to determine how best to promote optimal development.

Children transition to independent eating over the course of several years. *Jordan R. Green* and colleagues reviewed the development of chewing skills and factors affecting chewing, including food texture, feeding experience, and tooth emergence. They described studies into chewing motor development using biomechanical-based approaches that will add to our understanding of the oromotor control and coordination required to safely and efficiently learn to chew. Chewing development is an essential aspect of feeding readiness that is often not included in recommendations for complementary feeding, as little is known about the development of chewing motor skills and how children learn to accommodate to foods with varying textures. An understanding of these processes will enable advice related to provision of developmentally appropriate foods. Development of evidence-based guidelines regarding the safety and appropriateness of new foods will allow identification of children at risk for choking or feeding impairments, and will minimize feeding disorders.

As the prevalence of food allergies in many communities continues to rise, attention has turned to the role of common food allergens in allergy prevention strategies. The fourth speaker, *Debra J. Palmer* reviewed the most recent evidence related to complementary feeding and the development of allergy. Over recent years, several randomized controlled trials have been conducted to investigate the ideal age to introduce common allergens including peanut and egg into infant diets. To date the results from three of these trials have determined that there is no reason to delay the introduction of the common allergens into the infant's diet after solid foods have commenced. However, the trials have also highlighted the finding that some infants are sensitized to food allergens before they have ingested these foods. Thus, future research needs to focus on strategies to prevent early-life food allergen sensitization prior to complementary feeding.

Finally, *Erin S. Ross* discussed the development of taste and flavor preferences during infancy and later childhood, highlighting that food and eating is a sensory issue. The number of foods eaten as a young child has a strong influence on food diversity later in childhood. This is affected by the range of foods eaten by their parents, beginning with probable exposures to taste in utero. Flavor preferences affect the acceptance of novel foods, and infants and young children may require multiple tastes before they accept a food into their diet. With the introduction of both complementary and textured foods, infants develop preferences for foods. Learning to eat a new food is a developmental process, and offering repeated exposures is an effective way to teach children to eat more nutritious foods such as vegetables, but parents typically only offer foods 2–3 times before deciding if their child likes the food. While parents may use appropriate behaviors with a child who accepts most sensory inputs easily, they may resort to ineffective strategies with children who have challenges around accepting new foods. Strategies to help parents be more successful in achieving taste exposures in a positive social environment need to be identified.

In summary, the early feeding period is important for setting early taste preferences and has an important influence on long-term dietary patterns. In addition to underpinning nutritional status, good dietary variety may be helpful in preventing the development of food allergies and other noncommunicable diseases.

Maria Makrides

Black RE, Makrides M, Ong KK (eds): Complementary Feeding: Building the Foundations for a Healthy Life. Nestlé Nutr Inst Workshop Ser, vol 87, pp 63–72, (DOI: 10.1159/000448938)
Nestec Ltd., Vevey/S. Karger AG., Basel, © 2017

Patterns of Growth in Early Childhood and Infectious Disease and Nutritional Determinants

Robert E. Black

Bloomberg School of Public Health, Johns Hopkins University, Baltimore, MD, USA

Abstract

The physical growth of young children in low- and middle-income countries is reduced compared to international standards. The deviations in growth in both weight and height are greatest in the first 2 years of life and this has serious consequences for child mortality, development, adult stature, and health. The determinants of these patterns of growth faltering include intergenerational factors, such as maternal height, short birth interval, and conditions in pregnancy, including maternal underweight and anemia. These factors contribute to fetal growth restriction and premature delivery, which put many infants on a different growth trajectory. Postnatal exposure to microbes resulting in diarrhea and febrile infectious diseases and poor quality diet further compromise growth. Determinants of growth faltering after birth vary by setting and are not independent of each other. For example, the adverse effects of diarrhea on growth may be mitigated by a high-quality diet. Global estimates suggest that 25% of stunting can be attributed to fetal growth restriction and even more in countries in South Asia with a high prevalence of low birth weight. Infectious diseases may contribute a similar amount and subclinical enteric infections can result in intestinal dysfunction with adverse effects on nutrition and growth. Dietary factors, especially consumption of complementary foods of insufficient quality, have a paramount role in growth faltering in the critical period of infancy.

Introduction

Physical growth in infants and young children follows a predictable pattern consistent with internationally applicable standards for weight and length/height by age [1]. Inadequate weight gain or linear growth in early childhood is of concern in low- and middle-income countries (LMIC) because substantial deviations from the expected pattern are associated with increased disease burden and death from infections, impaired cognitive development, and adult metabolic disease [2]. Vice versa, inadequate growth increases or excessive weight gain is less of a problem in LMIC in young children, although rates of overweight in older children are increasing in some settings [2]; these issues will not be considered further in this paper.

The determinants of optimum growth in early childhood are multiple and occur at several levels [2]. At the most distal level, the socioeconomic and political context, undernutrition is associated with poverty and inequitable distribution of resources, and these are linked to an intermediate level of determinants. These include food insecurity with limited availability and economic access to food of sufficient quantity and quality, poor caregiving practices, and an unhygienic and unsafe environment. These intermediate-level conditions lead to a set of proximal determinants that have direct effects on child nutrition and development. Suboptimal breastfeeding, inadequate consumption of nutrient-rich foods, poor feeding practices, and high exposure to pathogenic microbes have direct consequences for child growth. In addition, there are intergenerational influences in which undernourished women have babies who have had growth restriction in utero with adverse health consequences after birth. These proximal determinants will be the focus of this paper.

Patterns of Growth in Low- and Middle-Income Countries

The nutritional anthropometric status is most often assessed by comparison of the child's measurements to the expected length/height or weight on the basis of the WHO Child Growth Standards [1]. Underweight is defined as having a weight2 z-scores below the median weight for that age and sex. Stunting is defined as having a length or height 2 z-scores below that expected for age and sex. Wasting is defined as having weight for a given length or height 2 scores below the median weight for length in the Growth Standards. Stunting is the most appropriate metric to reflect chronic undernutrition and wasting, and especially severe wasting (weight for length or height 3 z-scores below the median) is said to represent more acute malnutrition, although it is commonly found in

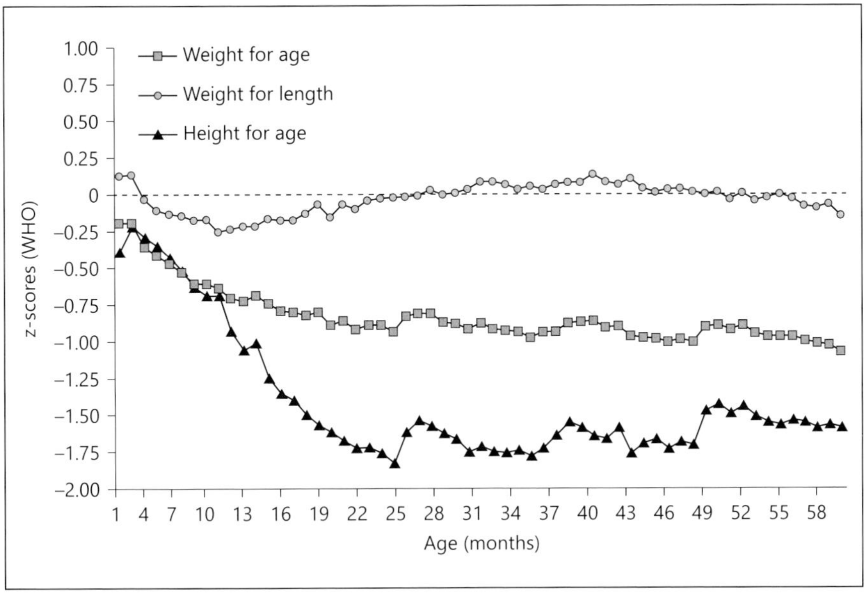

Fig. 1. Mean anthropometric z-scores according to age (1–59 months) for all 54 studies relative to the WHO standard. Reproduced with permission from *Pediatrics* [3] by the American Academy of Pediatrics.

populations with endemic food insecurity and not only in acute famine or emergency settings.

A comparison of anthropometric data from national surveys in LMIC with the WHO Child Growth Standards reveals some striking patterns [3]. In Asia, Africa, and the Americas the weight-for-age z-score starts in the first month of life near the standard median and declines progressively to about –1.0 weight-for-age z-score at 24 months of age (fig. 1). The height-for-age z-score below the standard in the first month then declines steeply to almost –2.0 z-scores and then increases slightly. Weight-for-height drops slightly below the standard in the first year of life and then returns to the expected value for the rest of childhood. These patterns differ markedly by world region. For height, the faltering of height-for-age z-score by 24 months of age is to about –1.0 for countries in the Americas, but to more than –2.0 for African and South Asian countries (fig. 2). Weight-for-height z-scores also vary greatly by region with values at or above the median of the standard except for South Asia with –0.75 to –1.0 from the first month of life throughout the first 5 years of life (fig. 3).

It has been estimated that in 2011 there were 165 million children with stunted linear growth, a decline from an estimated 253 million in 1990 [2]. The prevalence of stunting has declined from 40 to 26% in this period, an average annual rate of

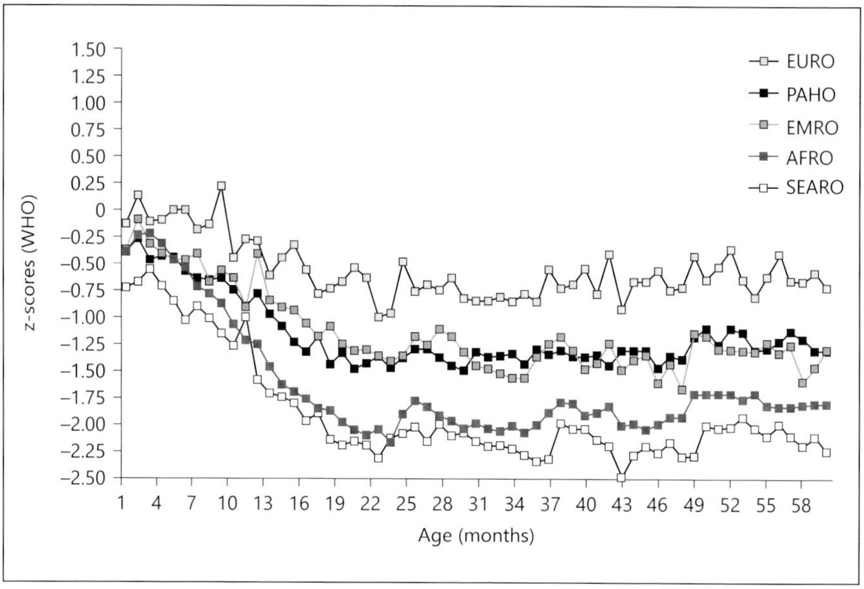

Fig. 2. Mean height-for-age z-scores by age (1–59 months) relative to the WHO standard according to region [Regional Offices for Africa (AFRO); the Eastern Mediterranean (EMRO); Europe (EURO); the Pan American Health Organization (PAHO), and Southeast Asia (SEARO)]. Reproduced with permission from *Pediatrics* [3] by the American Academy of Pediatrics.

reduction of about 2%. The highest prevalence estimates of approximately 40% are for South Asia and East and West Africa. With an increase in the number of children and the slowest regional decline in stunting prevalence, African countries have had an increase in the number of children with stunting while the numbers are declining in other world regions. Ninety percent of the stunted children in the world are in just 34 countries, nearly all in South Asia and sub-Saharan Africa.

The estimate for wasting in 2011 was 55 million children, a prevalence of 8% [2]. For 19 million children the wasting was severe (global prevalence of 3%); prevalences of 5–6% were found in South Asia and central Africa.

Determinants of Stunting

Numerous studies have identified important risk factors for linear growth faltering and stunting. Those identified in population cohorts from pregnancy to childhood include maternal conditions such as short stature (<160 cm), underweight (body mass index <18.5), maternal anemia (hemoglobin <110 g/l), age at delivery (<20 years), short birth interval (<2 years), and malaria. These risk

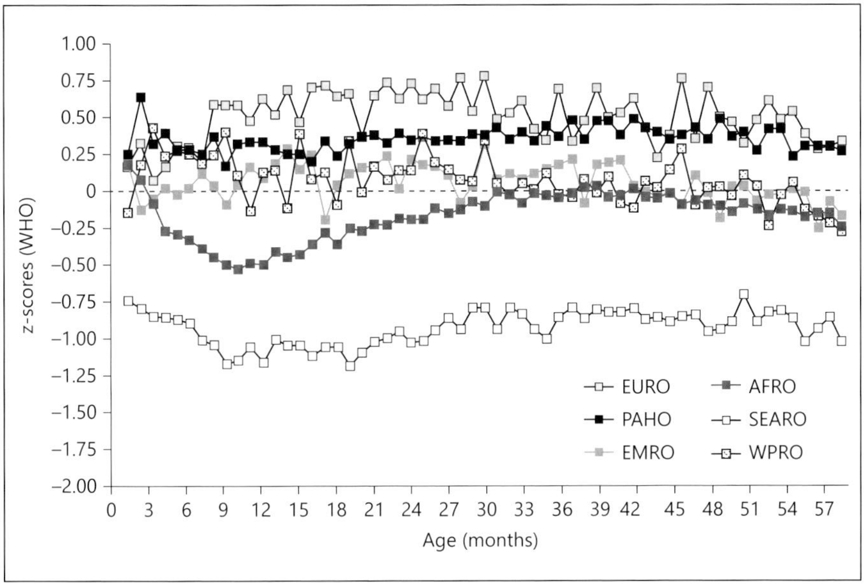

Fig. 3. Mean weight-for-height z-scores by age (1–59 months) relative to the WHO standard according to region [Regional Offices for Africa (AFRO); the Eastern Mediterranean (EMRO); Europe (EURO); Southeast Asia (SEARO); the Pan American Health Organization (PAHO), and the Western Pacific (WPRO)]. Reproduced with permission from *Pediatrics* [3] by the American Academy of Pediatrics.

factors are associated with fetal growth restriction and possibly preterm delivery, which put the newborn and infant on a different growth trajectory [2].

Fetal growth restriction and preterm birth have a broad set of determinants, including maternal and fetal infections, morbidity in pregnancy and placental insufficiency, smoking and indoor air pollution, drugs and alcohol, as well as underlying poverty [2]. This paper will not cover all of these factors, but will consider the importance of fetal growth restriction as assessed by the newborn being small for gestational age (SGA) based on comparison with well-off reference populations [4].

In 2010, an estimated 32 million babies were born SGA in LMIC – 27% of all live births [4]. The prevalence by world region varied widely from 7.0% in East to 25.5% in Sub-Saharan Africa and 44.5% in South Asia. Two thirds of SGA births are in Asia, with the highest prevalences and numbers in India and Pakistan. Babies who are SGA at birth have an elevated risk of mortality [2], and surviving infants have an increased rate of stunted linear growth. In comparison to births who were appropriate for gestational age and full-term, SGA full-term babies had increased odds of 2.4 of developing stunting by 24 months of age [5]. Babies with both SGA and preterm delivery had odds of 4.5 for later stunting. Similar increases in the odds of underweight and wasting were found for SGA births. Globally, 20% of stunting may be attributable to SGA, and in India and countries with a similarly high prevalence of SGA births, it is likely 35% or more [6].

For more than a half century, it has been understood that the frequent and sometimes severe infectious diseases affecting young children have adverse effects on growth and are important determinants of wasting and stunting [7]. For the former condition, the observation that severe illnesses such as measles can precipitate acute malnutrition and complications such as blindness from vitamin A deficiency provide an obvious link. For stunting, the observation of an association of frequent infectious diarrhea and respiratory disease episodes with growth faltering led to the studies that have tried to quantify the effects. In one analysis of pooled data from five LMIC, 25% of the stunting at 24 months of age was attributed to the child having five episodes of diarrhea in that time period [8]. These findings were unchanged by adjustment for socioeconomic status. There may be growth faltering during an episode of diarrhea but 'catch-up' growth after recovery when children grow more rapidly than previously. The magnitude of the effect of the illness and potential for catch-up are influenced by the child's age and pre-illness nutritional status, the etiology and severity of the illness, and both the duration of the illness and the subsequent illness-free period. There may also be an important relationship with the adequacy of the diet during and after the illness. Although it is recommended that during diarrhea children continue to be fed, there may be a reduction or alteration in the diet because of cultural beliefs or inappropriate medical advice [9]. If the usual diet consists of marginal calories and quality it may not allow more rapid catch up growth after illness. An illustration of the interaction of illness with diet is from a trial of food supplementation in children up to 36 months old in Colombia [10]. In the control group of children who did not receive the food supplement, there was a significant adverse effect on linear growth. However, in children who were routinely receiving the food supplements, there was no effect of diarrhea on growth. This effect modification of diarrhea by dietary adequacy was subsequently found in a secondary analysis of data from Guatemala [11]. This and other factors can explain the variation in the size of the effect of diarrhea on growth, although some effect is almost always found.

Effects of respiratory diseases and other febrile diseases on growth have been found but have been less consistent than for diarrhea and more difficult to quantify. However, there is increasing evidence for mechanisms by which such illnesses can have an effect through activation of an immune response and inflammation that have metabolic costs and may result in losses or shifts in micronutrients needed for growth [12]. These and other mechanisms may also occur with even subclinical infections. Of renewed interest in recent years is environmental enteric dysfunction (environmental enteropathy) [13, 14]. This is a condition characterized by abnormalities of the intestinal epithelium, altered barrier integrity, mucosal inflammation, and reduced nutrient absorption. This condition is likely due to the repeated ingestion of microorganisms beginning shortly after birth. The condition has been hypothesized to have adverse effects on growth that are yet to be quantified.

Diets that are inadequate in calories, protein, essential fatty acids, and micronutrients (essential vitamins and minerals) can result in poor growth. Breast milk is an important source of nutrients in the first months and years of life. Current recommendations are that babies be fed only breast milk for the first 6 months of life and that breastfeeding be continued along with complementary foods to at least the second birthday. Introduction of liquids or foods in the first 6 months can lead to a diet of reduced nutritional quality and exposure to microbes that can cause diarrhea and possibly environmental dysfunction. Failure to continue breastfeeding in the second half of infancy and feeding complementary foods of poor energy density and quality contribute to the faltering of both linear growth and weight gain in LMIC from 6 to about 24 months of age.

Observational studies of the determinants of stunting have shown significant relationships with reported food intake, as well as other factors. For example, a study in the Philippines found a positive effect of breastfeeding on linear growth, as well as negative influences of birth weight, diarrhea, and febrile respiratory diseases [15]. A study in Indonesia found positive effects on linear growth for the frequency of complementary food consumption, as well as maternal height and birth length [16]. In Bangladesh, there was less stunting in children having a more highly diverse diet, possibly reflecting better micronutrient intake [17].

Only one observational study had tried to compare the relative contributions of infectious diseases and low energy intake as assessed by quantification of dietary intake from in-home measurements of breastfeeding and complementary feeding in children 5–18 months of age in rural Bangladesh [18]. These children were ill with diarrhea on 11.0% of days and with a febrile illness on 8.7% of days. Their average caloric intake was only 70% of that recommended. The weight gain of these children was only 57% of that of the age- and sex-specific international reference population. It was calculated that the diarrhea and fever days explained 42% of the growth faltering and inadequate caloric intake the remaining 58%.

Intervention studies can also provide some quantification of the effects of infectious diseases and poor diet on growth. Studies of interventions to provide improved water, sanitation, and hygiene have had mixed results. Some trials assessing promotion of handwashing or provision of improved water supply, for example, found reduced rates of childhood diarrhea, but the limited studies available do not find a consistent effect on growth [19–21]. Trials of nutritional counseling regarding complementary feeding and/or provision of supplemental foods have shown benefits on growth [22] and will be reviewed in the paper by Dr. Heidkamp in this workshop series.

Of the many essential micronutrients [23], only zinc has been demonstrated to have an important role in physical growth. Severe zinc deficiency is associated with severe stunting, hypogonadism, and increased rates of infectious diseases, but is now rarely seen. However, inadequate zinc intake is highly prevalent in LMIC and is associated with poor growth in young children. The strongest evidence for this comes from many randomized controlled trials, and a meta-analysis of their results shows a statistically significant benefit of zinc supplementation on linear growth and stunting in preschool-age children [24, 25].

Conclusions

Growth in young children has intergenerational origins and multiple determinants. Maternal nutritional status, which is itself related to nutrition and growth from her childhood to childbearing years, is related to fetal growth and healthy development. From birth, babies may be on different growth trajectories determined by fetal growth restriction and preterm delivery. Globally, a quarter of stunting may be attributable to in utero conditions, and, in countries such as in South Asia with a high prevalence of low birth weight, this may increase to a third or more. The common infectious diseases of childhood also take a toll on growth. A quarter of stunting has been attributed to diarrhea, although this effect can be ameliorated by a high-quality diet. Oral exposure to microbes may result in alterations in the microbial flora and functions of the small bowel affecting growth even without diarrhea. Additional effects on growth are from febrile illnesses that have metabolic costs. Poor quality diets, with insufficient calories and essential macronutrients and micronutrients are likely the major determinant of poor growth in most LMIC. Efforts to reduce stunting and wasting will need to be multifaceted and include interventions in pregnancy and the first 2 years of life to address the infectious and dietary determinants of poor growth in this critical period and to provide the next generation with a better nutritional endowment [22].

Disclosure Statement

Dr. Black is a member of the Creating Shared Value Advisory Counsel of the Nestle Co. and is on the governing boards of the Micronutrient Initiative and Vitamin Angels.

References

1 WHO Multicentre Growth Reference Study Group: WHO Child Growth Standards based on length/height, weight and age. Acta Paediatr Suppl 2006;450:76–85.
2 Black RE, Victora CG, Walker SP, et al: Maternal and child undernutrition and overweight in low-income and middle-income countries. Lancet 2013;382:427–451.
3 Victora CG, de Onis M, Hallal PC, et al: Worldwide timing of growth faltering: revisiting implications for interventions. Pediatrics 2010;125:e473–e480.
4 Lee AC, Katz J, Blencowe H, et al: National and regional estimates of term and preterm babies born small for gestational age in 138 low-income and middle-income countries in 2010. Lancet Glob Health 2013;1:e26–e36.
5 Christian P, Lee SE, Donahue Angel M, et al: Risk of childhood undernutrition related to small-for-gestational age and preterm birth in low- and middle-income countries. I J Epidemiol 2013;42:1340–1355.
6 Black RE: Foetal growth restriction: nutritional determinants, consequences in children, and interventions. NFI Bulletin 2014; 35:1–5.
7 Scrimshaw NS, Taylor CE, Gordon JE: Interactions of nutrition and infection. Monogr Ser World Health Organ 1968;57: 3–329.
8 Checkley W, Buckley G, Gilman RH, et al: Multi-country analysis of the effects of diarrhoea on childhood stunting. Int J Epidemiol 2008;37:816–830.
9 Brown KH: Dietary management of acute childhood diarrhea: optimal timing of feeding and appropriate use of milks and mixed diets. J Pediatr 1991;118:S92–S98.
10 Lutter C, Mora J, Habicht JP, et al: Nutritional supplementation: effects on child stunting because of diarrhea. Am J Clin Nutr 1989;50: 1–8.
11 Lutter CK, Habicht J-P, Rivera JA, et al: The relationship between energy intake and diarrheal disease in their effects on child growth: biological model, evidence, and implications for public health policy. Food Nutr Bull 1992; 14:36–42.
12 Ahmed T, Auble D, Berkley JA, et al: An evolving perspective about the origins of childhood undernutrition and nutritional interventions that includes the gut microbiome. Ann NY Acad Sci 2014;1332:22–38.
13 Keusch GT, Denno DM, Black RE, et al: Environmental enteric dysfunction: pathogenesis, diagnosis, and clinical consequences. Clin Infect Dis 2014;59(suppl 4):S207–S212.
14 Keusch GT, Rosenberg IH, Denno DM, et al: Implications of acquired environmental enteric dysfunction for growth and stunting in infants and children living in low- and middle-income countries. Food Nutr Bull 2013; 34:357–364.
15 Adair LS, Guilkey DK: Age-specific determinants of stunting in Filipino children. J Nutr 1997;127:314–320.
16 Schmidt MK, Muslimatun S, West CE, et al: Nutritional status and linear growth of Indonesian infants in West Java are determined more by prenatal environment than by postnatal factors. J Nutr 2002;132:2202–2207.
17 Rah J, Akhter N, Semba R, et al: Low dietary diversity is a predictor of child stunting in rural Bangladesh. Eur J Clin Nutr 2010;64: 1393–1398.
18 Becker S, Black RE, Brown KH: Relative effects of diarrhea, fever, and dietary energy intake on weight gain in rural Bangladeshi children. Am J Clin Nutr 1991;53:1499–1503.
19 Clasen T, Boisson S, Routray P, et al: Effectiveness of a rural sanitation programme on diarrhoea, soil-transmitted helminth infection, and child malnutrition in Odisha, India: a cluster-randomised trial. Lancet Glob Health 2014;2:e645–e653.
20 Dangour AD, Watson L, Cumming O, et al: Interventions to improve water quality and supply, sanitation and hygiene practices, and their effects on the nutritional status of children. Cochrane Database Syst Rev 2013; 8:CD009382.
21 Pickering AJ, Djebbari H, Lopez C, et al: Effect of a community-led sanitation intervention on child diarrhoea and child growth in rural Mali: a cluster-randomised controlled trial. Lancet Glob Health 2015;3:e701–e711.
22 Bhutta ZA, Das JK, Rizvi A, et al: Evidence-based interventions for improvement of maternal and child nutrition: what can be done and at what cost? Lancet 2013;382:452–477.
23 Ruel-Bergeron JC, Stevens GA, Sugimoto JD, et al: Global update and trends of hidden hunger, 1995–2011: the hidden hunger index. PLoS One 2015;10:e0143497.

24 Brown KH, Peerson JM, Rivera J, et al: Effect of supplemental zinc on the growth and serum zinc concentrations of prepubertal children: a meta-analysis of randomized controlled trials. Am J Clin Nutr 2002;75: 1062–1071.

25 Imdad A, Bhutta ZA: Effect of preventive zinc supplementation on linear growth in children under 5 years of age in developing countries: a meta-analysis of studies for input to the lives saved tool. BMC Public Health 2011;11(suppl 3):S22.

Black RE, Makrides M, Ong KK (eds): Complementary Feeding: Building the Foundations for a Healthy Life. Nestlé Nutr Inst Workshop Ser, vol 87, pp 73–87, (DOI: 10.1159/000448939)
Nestec Ltd., Vevey/S. Karger AG., Basel, © 2017

Measuring Infant and Young Child Complementary Feeding Practices: Indicators, Current Practice, and Research Gaps

Marie T. Ruel

International Food Policy Research Institute, Washington, DC, USA

Abstract

The publication of the WHO Infant and Young Child Feeding (IYCF) indicators in 2008 equipped the nutrition and broader development community with an invaluable tool for measuring, documenting, and advocating for faster progress in improving these practices in low- and middle-income countries (LMICs). The indicators, with 5 of them focusing on complementary feeding (CF) practices, were originally designed for population level assessment, targeting, monitoring, and evaluation. This chapter takes stock of where we are with the existing CF indicators: it reviews how the indicators have been used, what we have learned, and what their strengths and limitations are, and it suggests a way forward. We find that the indicators have been used extensively for population level assessments and country comparisons, and to track progress. They have also been adopted by researchers in program impact evaluations and in research seeking to understand the determinants and consequences of poor CF practices for child growth and development outcomes. In addition to generating a wealth of knowledge and unveiling the severity of the global problem of poor CF practices in LMICs, the indicators have been an invaluable tool to raise awareness and call for urgent action on improving CF practices at scale. The indicators have strengths and limitations, which are summarized in this chapter. Although enormous progress has been achieved since the indicators were released in 2008, we feel it is time to reflect and revisit the CF indicators, improve them, develop new ones, and promote their appropriate use. Better indicators are critically important to stimulate action and investments in improving CF practices at scale.

Introduction

The publications *Guiding Principles for Complementary Feeding of the Breastfed Child* [1] and *Guiding Principles for Feeding Non-Breastfed Children* [2], and the subsequent development of a set of indicators to measure Infant and Young Child Feeding (IYCF) practices [3] were critical milestones for improving awareness and stimulating programmatic and policy action to improve IYCF practices globally. Since their release, the WHO IYCF indicators have indeed been used extensively for population level assessments and national or regional comparisons, as well as for program design, targeting, monitoring, and evaluation, and for tracking global progress. The indicators have also been used widely for research aimed at understanding the determinants of IYCF practices and to document associations between IYCF practices and child nutrition, health, and development outcomes. As is widely recognized, having indicators to measure a given construct is critically important for raising its profile as well as for advocacy and for fostering the policy dialogue. The IYCF indicators were no exception, and their release has equipped the nutrition community with an invaluable tool for measuring, documenting, and advocating for faster progress in improving IYCF practices in low- and middle-income countries (LMICs).

The aim of this chapter is to take stock of where we are with the existing set of IYCF indicators; it reviews how they have been used, what we have learned, and what their strengths and limitations are, and suggests a way forward. Consistent with the overall theme of this book, the focus is on indicators of *complementary feeding* (CF) practices; indicators of breastfeeding practices are not discussed. The chapter is organized as follows: first we review the status of the existing set of indicators of CF practices; second we present a brief overview of how and for what purposes the indicators have been used and summarize key findings, and third we discuss the strengths and limitations of the indicators and conclude with suggestions for the way forward.

What Is the Status of the Existing Set of Indicators of Complementary Feeding Practices?

The WHO indicators for assessing IYCF practices include 8 core indicators, of which 3 are focused on breastfeeding and 5 on CF practices [3]. The additional 7 optional indicators measure different aspects of breastfeeding. Thus, a total of 5 indicators are available for the measurement of CF practices. The indicators are listed in box 1, along with a short description of the key dimension of CF practices they are meant to measure.

Box 1. List of WHO indicators of CF and the key dimensions they are meant to measure [3]

1 Introduction of solid, semi-solid, and soft foods: optimal timing of introduction of complementary foods (CFo)
2 Minimum dietary diversity (MDD): micronutrient adequacy of the diet (diet quality)
3 Minimum meal frequency (MMF): energy adequacy of the diet (quantity of food)
4 Minimum acceptable diet (MAD): composite indicator combining breastfeeding and CF indicators 2 and 3
5 Consumption of iron-rich and iron-fortified foods: adequacy of iron intake

The IYCF indicators were developed using an extensive, multi-stakeholder consultative process [4] that relied on the available guiding principles for feeding breastfed [1] or nonbreastfed children 6–24 months of age [2]. The guiding principles, in turn, were developed through a series of technical consultations and relied on available evidence at the time regarding the nutritional needs of healthy infants and young children living in the developing world. The result was a set of 10 guiding principles for the breastfed child and 9 for the nonbreastfed child. The guiding principles include recommendations related to exclusive breastfeeding for the first 6 months; continued breastfeeding for up to 24 months or beyond (these first 2 recommendations are omitted in the guidance for the nonbreastfed child); the timely introduction and feeding of adequate foods in the right amount and the right quality, texture, and safety, and appropriate feeding during illnesses (table 1, left column) for guiding principles for the breastfed child).

When designing the IYCF indicators, a main consideration was that the indicators were to be used in large surveys for population assessments, and, therefore, they had to be simple and practical, yet valid and reliable [4]. This consideration limited the number of dimensions of optimal CF practices that could be captured in the set of indicators; for example, aspects such as responsive feeding, age-specific texture of food, food safety, and appropriate feeding during illnesses are not easily amenable to recall-, survey-based methods of measurement. As a result, the set of WHO indicators of CF practices measures only a subset of the multiple dimensions of optimal feeding represented in the guiding principles. Table 1 illustrates this point; it presents a summary of the 10 guiding principles for complementary feeding of the breastfed child and highlights which of the guiding principles have a corresponding indicator to measure it. Of the 8 guiding principles related to CF practices, only 4 have a corresponding indicator in the WHO set of core indicators [timing, energy (quantity), diversity (quality), and iron-rich foods]. The 5th WHO indicator of CF practices is a composite indicator, which combines information on current breastfeeding, meal frequency, and dietary diversity (DD). This shows that the set of indicators currently available for measuring CF practices covers only a subset of all essential behaviors that comprise optimal complementary feeding practices.

Table 1. The 10 *guiding principles* for complementary feeding of the breastfed child and related WHO indicators

Guiding principles/dimension of child feeding	Recommended practice	WHO indicator?	
	Recommendation	Yes	No
Duration of exclusive breastfeeding (EBF) and timing of introduction of CFo	EBF up to 6 months Introduction of CFo at 6 months	EBF Introduction of solid, semi-solid or soft foods	
Maintenance of BF	Continue frequent, on-demand BF up to 2 years of age or beyond	Continued BF at 1 year	
Responsive feeding	Practice responsive feeding		X
Safe preparation and storage of CFo			X
Amount of CFo	Energy needs for BF infant: 6–8 months: 200 kcal 9–11 months: 300 kcal 12–23 months: 550 kcal		X
Food consistency	Increase food consistency and variety as infant gets older		X
Meal frequency/energy density	Increase number of times child is fed CFo with age. Number of feedings depends on energy density. Recommended: 6–8 months: 2–3 times/day 9–24 months: 3–4 times/day Add nutritious snacks	Minimum meal frequency (MMF)	
Nutrient content of CFo	Feed variety of foods to ensure nutrient needs are met. Meat, poultry, fish, eggs should be eaten daily or as often as possible; adequate fat content needed	Minimum dietary diversity (MDD)	
Use of vitamin-mineral supplement or fortified products for infant and mother		Consumption of iron-rich and iron-fortified food	
Feeding during and after illness			X

How Has the Current Set of Indicators of CF Practices Been Used So Far?

The WHO indicators of CF practices were designed as population level indicators to be used primarily for assessment, population targeting, and monitoring and evaluation. They have been used for all these purposes. In addition, they have also been used by researchers to explore the determinants of CF practices as well as for analyzing the associations between CF practices and child health and nutrition outcomes. A brief summary of how the indicators have been used so far for some of these purposes is provided below.

Population Level Assessment and Country Comparisons
One of the first uses of the new indicators was the development of 'country profiles' which were published as part 3 of the series on *Indicators for Assessing Infant and Young Child Feeding Practices* [5]. Nationally representative data from the Demographic and Health Surveys (DHS) (2002–2008) for 46 countries were used to create country profiles of IYCF practices using 13 of the 15 indicators. Data to construct the indicators were already available in DHS prior to the publication of the WHO indicators for 13 of the 15 indicators (7 core and 6 optional indicators; data were unavailable for consumption of iron-rich foods and for milk feeding for nonbreastfed children). The findings revealed grossly inadequate CF practices in most of the countries, and especially in sub-Saharan Africa and South Asia. Minimum DD (MDD) was particularly low across countries in these regions, and, in sub-Saharan Africa, all countries had less than 30% of children achieving minimum acceptable diets (MAD). A similar exercise was carried out in 2014 using DHS data (2005–2013) from 37 LMICs from sub-Saharan Africa, Asia, and Latin America [6]. A similar pattern to the one described in 2010 emerged, where few countries had more than 30% of children achieving MDD and only one (Indonesia) had more than 30% achieving the MAD. The analysis went further and examined differences in CF practices by subgroup and found marked differences, with children faring better if they were older, lived in urban compared to rural areas, had a more educated mother, and lived in a wealthier household. A pooled analysis of data from 46 DHS surveys (2002–2008) confirmed the poor state of CF practices globally (in LMICs), with less than one third of children meeting MDD, approximately half meeting the minimum number of meals of complementary foods (CFo) per day, and only 21% achieving MAD [7]. Consistent with previous findings, Africa and Asia fared much worse on all 3 indicators than Latin America.

Overall, these first population level data on CF practices were critically important to unveil the severity of the global problem of poor IYCF practices in LMICs, and the WHO indicators were an invaluable tool to help documentation, raise awareness, and call for urgent action on solving the problem.

Monitoring and Evaluation of Programs and Interventions Aimed at Improving Infant and Young Child Feeding Practices
Most of the reviews of the impacts of programs aimed at improving IYCF practices have traditionally focused on impacts on child growth, morbidity, or

development outcomes, rather than on how the interventions changed the practices that might have translated into changes in child outcomes [8–10]. A recent systematic review including 16 studies documents an impact of education and interventions to improve complementary feeding on the uptake of recommended foods [11], recognizing that changes in practices are likely to be part of the pathway to improved child anthropometry. It is likely, however, that one of the reasons why impacts on CF practices have not been documented in past reviews of education programs was the absence of standard indicators to facilitate comparison. The availability of the WHO IYCF indicators has helped change this pattern and several ongoing or recent evaluations of nutrition-sensitive programs that include a behavior change communication (BCC) strategy are specifically measuring improvements in IYCF practices as an impact indicator, in addition to child growth and development outcomes. Findings from the Alive and Thrive project, for example, document meaningful impacts of social media and interpersonal communication on several CF practices in Bangladesh and Vietnam [12]. Similarly, a nutrition-sensitive agriculture and nutrition and health BCC program targeted at women in Burkina Faso shows an increase in the percentage of children who achieved MDD among program participants compared to children from the control group, and at end line, children who had consumed ≥4 food groups in the previous 24 h were more likely to have consumed nutrient-rich foods than those who had not achieved MDD [13]. The authors noted that greater diversity and quality of CFo among study participants are likely to be part of the pathway of impacts found on child morbidity, wasting, and anemia.

The recent shift in the measurement and reporting of changes in IYCF practices in the context of research and impact evaluations is likely due to the availability of a new set of standard indicators that facilitates measurement and comparison across studies. Also, with the national level statistics and country profiles highlighting how dire the situation is with respect to child feeding in LMICs, countries and programs are increasingly taking action to improve IYCF as a key outcome of its own and eager to document progress.

Understanding the Associations between Complementary Feeding Practices and Child Anthropometry

Child DD scores have been developed and used as a proxy for dietary quality to look at associations with child anthropometric outcomes since the late 1990s, several years before the WHO indicators were released (summarized by Ruel [14]). In a parallel process, DD indicators for infants and young children 6–23 months of age were validated through a multicountry study, to assess their performance in predicting dietary quality, defined as the mean probability of adequacy of 9 key micronutrients in CFo [15]. The validation, which used 10 data sets from countries in Africa, Asia, and Latin America, informed the development of the WHO 7-food group DD indicator, and the selection of the cutoff point (≥4 food groups) for the MDD indicator was based on the study results and subsequent stakeholder consultations.

The positive association between DD indicators and child anthropometry has been documented through several studies conducted in a variety of contexts and using different approaches, measurement tools, and indicators. Overall, the associations are robust and remain after controlling for potentially confounding factors such as energy intake and sociodemographic and economic factors [16]. Associations are consistently found for linear growth (height-for-age z-score), and in some cases they are also documented for weight-for-height and weight-for-age z-scores. The findings and details of these studies are summarized by Ruel [14] and Ruel et al. [16].

More recently, studies have examined the associations between the broader set of IYCF indicators and child anthropometry. A pooled analysis of 14 DHS data sets (2003–2006) from Africa and South Asia shows that, among infants 6–8 months of age, consumption of solid foods was associated with a lower risk of both stunting and underweight [17]. In their model for children 6–23 months of age, meeting MDD, consuming iron-rich foods, and achieving minimum acceptable diet (MAD) were also associated with a lower risk of both stunting and underweight, whereas consuming the minimum number of meals recommended was associated with a lower probability of underweight only. A review of 8 studies that examined country-specific associations between IYCF indicators and child anthropometry showed, again, a positive association between DD and height-for-age z-score in 3 of the countries (Bangladesh, India, and Zambia) and an association with MAD in 4 countries (the same three and Ethiopia) [18]. Complementary feeding indicators were not associated with weight-for-height z-scores, with the exception of minimum meal frequency (MMF) in one country (Uganda), and associations with stunting or wasting were generally not statistically significant. No associations were found between consumption of iron-rich foods and child anthropometry in any of the 5 countries for which data were available.

A special journal issue focused on complementary feeding practices in South Asia includes a series of papers presenting descriptive analyses of patterns of CF practices in five countries and detailed analyses of their determinants [19]. The comparative analysis results show that low education and socioeconomic status are key determinants of poor CF practices in the region; other factors include the limited exposure to media, inadequate antenatal care, and the limited postnatal contacts between mothers and health staff [20].

Clearly, the WHO IYCF indicators have been used extensively to address important gaps in our knowledge and understanding of patterns, and determinants and consequences of poor child feeding practices. As noted by Jones et al. [18], however, for these more refined, individual (as opposed to population) level analyses aimed at characterizing the contribution of child food and nutrition intake and feeding practices to improving child nutritional status in specific contexts, additional indicators and more precise measures may be needed.

What Are the Strengths and Limitations of the 2008 WHO Complementary Feeding Indicators?

The WHO 2008 document describes how the IYCF (including the CF) indicators should be used and what some of their limitations are. The key points are the following:

1 the indicators were meant to be simple and practical, yet valid and reliable;

2 they were designed to be used for population level assessments, targeting, monitoring, and evaluation;

3 they focus on selected food-related aspects of child feeding, which are amenable to population level assessment;

4 they were designed to be used in large-scale surveys; for some indicators that are age specific and focus on small age ranges, e.g. exclusive breastfeeding (0–6 months) and timely introduction of CFo (6–8 months), sample sizes may be too small for using in smaller local data collection exercises, and

5 they were meant to be used together (as a full set of indicators) because of the multidimensional nature of appropriate infant and young child feeding.

The previous section showed that since their release, the IYCF (and CF) indicators have been used extensively for most of the purposes for which they were originally designed, especially for population level assessment, country comparisons and monitoring global trends, and for program monitoring and evaluation. They have been very useful for these purposes and have been instrumental in raising awareness among a wide range of stakeholders and highlighting the need for immediate action to improve IYCF practices at scale.

The indicators, however, have been used for purposes that go beyond their original intent, especially the extensive association research that explores the household, maternal and child determinants of CF practices, and the associations between CF practices and child outcomes. The indicators, which were originally designed for population level assessment, may be of limited usefulness for individual level association analyses. The multiple potential sources of measurement error that affect proxy indicators such as the WHO CF practices indicators may indeed result in attenuation of the magnitude and statistical significance of the associations hypothesized (due to misclassification). The inconsistent results found in multicountry analyses of the associations between CF indicators and child anthropometry, for example, likely reflect this problem. Moreover, the association research carried out so far has been done separately for each indicator, which violates the recommendation to use the full set of indicators for meaningful interpretation. Indeed, what matters for child nutrition and health is the quality of all CF practices over time, but multivariate analysis models using cross-sectional data only analyze one practice at a time at one specific point in time and therefore fail to capture the cumulative long-term effects of the compendium of CF practices on child outcomes.

Overall, the WHO CF indicators may be appropriate when rough proxies of the quality of CF practices are needed, but are likely to lack specificity and precision for more refined analyses such as association studies or causal mediation analyses to model pathways of associations or impacts of interventions, which require more precise indicators.

Table 2 presents an overview of the 5 CF indicators and highlights some of the measurement and validation issues that may affect their usefulness for certain purposes. The key issues are discussed briefly below.

Validation against a Gold Standard

As seen in table 2, only 1 of the 5 CF indicators has been properly validated against a gold standard representing the construct that the indicator is meant to reflect. As noted in section 3c, the DD indicator was validated through an extensive multicountry analysis using a standard methodology and was determined to be strongly associated with the mean micronutrient adequacy of CFo in all the data sets analyzed. None of the other indicators was validated through a rigorous analysis to assess performance in predicting the underlying construct intended.

Likely to Reflect an Underlying Construct?

An issue related to the lack of validation of the indicators is the question of whether or not they are likely to reflect the underlying construct they are intended to measure. The indicator on *introduction of CFo* measures the percent of children 6–8 months of age who were fed CFo in the previous 24 h. This indicator therefore informs us of whether or not children in this age group are actually receiving CFo, but it does not inform us of whether the introduction of CFo was indeed timely (between 6 and 8 months). As defined, the in-

Table 2. Summary of measurement issues related to the 5 WHO indicators of CF practices (using the indicators for breastfed children only)

Indicator	Introduction of solid, semi-solid or soft foods	Minimum dietary diversity (MDD)	Minimum meal frequency (MMF)	Minimum acceptable diet (MAD)	Consumption of iron-rich or iron-fortified foods
Definition	% 6–8 months old who received in previous 24 h	% 6–23 months who received foods from 4+ groups in past 24 h	% 6–23 months who received CFo minimum number of times (≥2 for 6–8 months; ≥for 9–23 months) in past 24 h	Index combining 3 recommended practices (BF, MDD and MMF)	% 6–23 months old who consumed iron-rich food, iron-fortified special food or home fortificants
Aimed to measure which dimension of complementary feeding?	Appropriate timing of introduction of CFo	Micronutrient adequacy of CFo	Energy adequacy of CFo, assuming adequate energy density of diet	Combined index of adequacy of 3 recommended IYCF practices	Intake of (bioavailable) iron
Indicator validated? If so, against what?	No	Yes, in different contexts, for micronutrient adequacy of 9 essential micronutrients; not validated for essential fatty acids	No	No	No
Likely to represent underlying construct?	Does not capture too early (<6 months) or very late (≥9 months) introduction; only late (6–8 months)	Yes, robust, but also associated with energy intake and socioeconomic status measures of well-being	Unclear (given issues related to energy density, difficulties differentiating snacks from meals, and identifying which feeding episodes count as a meal)	Unclear; limited to 3 dimensions of CF practices	Yes, if iron-rich foods, iron-fortified special foods, and home fortificants available in survey area are well identified prior to survey and their iron content is documented
Subject to recall error or bias?	Yes	Yes	Yes	Yes	Yes
Other key measurement challenges	Introduction of CFo can be very gradual; indicator does not capture timing of regular feeding of CFo, nor very small amounts of food consumed	Prone to errors and misclassification due small amounts consumed; does not reflect usual diet	Prone to errors and misclassification due to small amounts of food consumed and other factors listed above; does not reflect usual diet	Limitations of indices that combine different indicators (does not provide information on individual components)	Prone to errors and misclassification due to small amounts consumed; does not reflect usual diet
Likely to reflect usual or long-term practice?	No	No	No	No	No

dicator fails to detect the problems of early introduction of CFo (<6 months) or very late introduction (≥9 months), which limits its overall usefulness. As noted above, the *MDD* indicator has been properly validated and shown to accurately reflect the micronutrient adequacy of the diet, an indicator of dietary quality. The indicator on *MMF* is meant to be used as a rough proxy for energy intake from CFo and relies on the critically important assumption that the energy density of CFo is adequate [1, 2]. In large surveys, as well as in more focused impact evaluation surveys, it has proven almost impossible to assess the mean energy density of CFo, and even if it was possible, adjustments would need to be made by expert nutritionists to decide what cutoff points to use for different age groups when energy density is lower than recommended. The other difficulty related to data collection is distinguishing between meals and snacks, and the challenge of clearly identifying which feeding episodes count for a meal. These data collection challenges are likely to make this indicator particularly prone to measurement errors and misclassification, and may make the indicator a relatively poor proxy for energy intake. The *MAD* is a composite index that includes 3 dimensions of CF practices (continued breastfeeding, *MDD*, and *MMF*). As such, the indicator is not expected to reflect the complexity of all aspects that encompass optimal CF practices, but it can be a good summary of the 3 domains it aims to capture. The *consumption of iron-rich or iron-fortified foods* is a straightforward indicator that has the potential to accurately reflect the child's intake of iron in the previous 24 h. The key issue that determines the usefulness of the indicator in this case is data collection practice, which requires that field workers have a complete list and iron content of all foods and products that are either iron rich or iron fortified, and that they probe adequately to get the name and brand of each one of them, and record label information for the products that are not on the list.

Recall Error and Bias

All indicators are collected through 24-hour recall methods. This approach is known to lead to possible *recall error* (random error due to poor memory) or to *recall bias*, which is particularly problematic when respondents have been exposed to education/BCC campaigns aimed at improving the practices of interest and are aware of what the desired responses are. This makes the indicators particularly susceptible to systematic overestimation of impacts in studies measuring the impact of education campaigns on CF practices. Social desirability assessment is one method that has been used to assess whether recall bias might be a problem in a given population [12], but the approach does not provide a way to correct for it where the problem exists.

Other Key Measurement Challenges
The indicator on *introduction of CFo* takes a snapshot of whether or not a child has consumed semi-solid or solid foods in the previous 24 h. The hypothesis is that yesterday is a good reflection of *usual* practice, when in fact it is well known that consumption of CFo in young infants is a dynamic process that may vary from day to day until feeding becomes more established. The proxy indicator cannot reflect on the timing of regular intake of CFo by the infant. The same is true for the other indicators, which capture practice in the past 24 h but not usual practice. All 4 indicators also suffer from an additional measurement challenge: that of not capturing small amounts consumed, which is common in young children, and leads to overestimation of adequate practice. For MAD, the problem often highlighted for composite indices is that they do not reflect the individual components that they include. This is not a problem in this case because the indicator is usually presented along with the other indicators that are included in the composite index.

Finally, the set of WHO indicators was originally developed to capture a few select dimensions of optimal infant and young child feeding practices, with a focus on preventing and reducing childhood undernutrition. The guiding principles as well as the indicators did not include considerations specific to the prevention of childhood (and related lifelong) overweight and obesity, a problem rapidly emerging even in LMICs [21].

Way Forward

This brief overview of the state, use, and strengths and weaknesses of the WHO CF indicators brings us to two main conclusions. First, in their 8 years of existence, the indicators have made tremendous contributions to enhancing awareness and knowledge about the status of CF practices nationally and globally. This has stimulated unprecedented interest and commitment among nutritionists and the wider development community to renew efforts to tackle the neglected area of CF practices as one of the critical inputs to accelerating progress in improving child nutrition. Second, the indicators have been used successfully for all the purposes for which they were originally designed, including population level assessments, tracking trends, and progress, and for program monitoring and evaluation. They have also been used extensively for research purposes, especially for individual level association analyses aimed at deepening our understanding of the determinants and consequences of CF practices and guide action to improve them. The use of the indicators in association research, however, has brought to light some of the key limitations of the indicators and the need to revisit available tools and measurement approaches. The indicators were originally designed to serve as rough proxies for a few CF behaviors that were amenable to being measured in large-scale data collection exercises; they were not designed to provide in-depth understanding of the intricacies and complexities of the multiple dimensions of CF practices or to describe usual practices at different ages.

The time has come to revisit how we can improve our measurement of CF practices and enhance our set of indicators. Initially, this exercise could include the following next steps:

- revisit the existing set of indicators and carry out validation studies, especially for indicators such as introduction of CFo, MMF and consumption of iron-rich and iron-fortified foods to assess whether or not the indicators accurately reflect the constructs they are meant to measure;
- as part of the validation exercises, assess whether or not the underlying assumptions (e.g., adequate energy density, snacks, and meals properly differentiated, foods consumed in small amounts not included) are adequate and develop simple ways to verify the assumptions and adjust the indicators accordingly in data collection procedures;
- assess the magnitude of error associated with the use of recall methods (with and without exposure to nutrition/BCC intervention);
- revisit the guiding principles and determine whether other dimensions of CF practices could be added to the set of indicators using innovative tools, technologies, and methods. Of particular importance would be the development of simple indicators to measure responsive feeding, feeding during and after illnesses, and safety in the preparation and storage of food;
- develop a simplified, technology-smart 24-hour dietary assessment method to quantitatively measure nutrient intake in children 6–24 months of age, for use in research or relatively small scale data collection exercises (including program impact evaluations), and
- develop and validate new indicators to reflect optimal practices for the prevention of childhood overweight and obesity.

Measuring complementary feeding practices is particularly complex given the series of practices and dimensions that comprise optimal practices; the fact that practices are highly dynamic and expected to change rapidly within short time frames, and the fact that breast milk intake varies widely between and within children thereby affecting their nutrient needs from CFo. Survey tools such as the WHO CF indicators can only provide a snapshot of current practices at a given age; they are not designed to capture the dynamic nature and interdependence of multiple practices over time. Research, however, could shed light on these processes by using more sophisticated tools and indicators and following cohorts of children over time. This type of research could be particularly useful to guide future efforts to enhance the range and performance of our indicators of CF practices.

Enormous progress has been achieved in measuring and understanding CF practices since the release of the WHO IYCF indicators in 2008. It is now time to reflect and revisit our indicators, improve them, develop new ones, and promote their appropriate use. Better indicators are critically important to stimulate action and investments in improving CF practices at scale.

Disclosure Statement

The author declares that no financial or other conflict of interest exists in relation to the content of the chapter.

References

1 Pan American Health Organization /World Health Organization: Guiding Principles for Complementary Feeding of the Breastfed Child. Washington, Pan American Health Organization/ WHO, 2003.

2 World Health Organization: Guiding Principles for Feeding Non-Breastfed Children 6–24 Months of Age. Geneva, WHO, 2005.

3 World Health Organization: Indicators for Assessing Infant and Young Child Feeding Practices. Part 1: Definitions. Geneva, WHO, 2008.

4 Arimond M, Daelmans B, Dewey K: Indicators for feeding practices in children. Lancet 2008;371:541–542.

5 World Health Organization: Indicators for Assessing Infant and Young Child Feeding Practices. Part 3: Country Profiles. Geneva, WHO, 2010.

6 Kothari MT, Abderrahim N, Coile A, Cheng Y: Nutritional Status of Women and Children. Rockville, ICF International, 2014.

7 Lutter CK, Daelmans BMEG, de Onis M, et al: Undernutrition, poor feeding practices, and low coverage of key nutrition interventions. Pediatrics, 2011, http://pediatrics.aappublications.org/content/early/2011/11/04/peds.2011-1392.abstract.

8 Caulfield LE, Huffman SL, Piwoz E: Interventions to improve intake of complementary foods by infants 6 to 12 months of age in developing countries: impact on growth and on the prevalence of malnutrition and potential contribution to child survival. Food Nutr Bull 1999;20:183–200.

9 Dewey KG, Adu-Afarwuah S: Systematic review of the efficacy and effectiveness of complementary feeding interventions in developing countries. Matern Child Nutr 2008; 24–85, http://onlinelibrary.wiley.com/doi/10.1111/j.1740–8709.2007.00124.x/full.

10 Imdad A, Yakoob MY, Bhutta Z: Impact of maternal education about complementary feeding and provision of complementary foods on child growth in developing countries. BMC Public Health 2011;11(suppl 3): S25.

11 Lassi ZS, Das JK, Zahid G, et al: Impact of education and provision of complementary feeding on growth and morbidity in children less than 2 years of age in developing countries: a systematic review. BMC Public Health 2013;13(suppl 3):S13.

12 Menon P, Nguyen PH, Saha KK, et al: Impacts on breastfeeding practices of at-scale strategies that combine intensive interpersonal counseling, mass media, and community mobilization: results of cluster-randomized program evaluations in Bangladesh and Viet Nam. PLoS Med 2016;13:e1002159.
13 Olney DK, Pedehombga A, Ruel MT, Dillon A: A 2-year integrated agriculture and nutrition and health behavior change communication program targeted to women in Burkina Faso reduces anemia, wasting, and diarrhea in children 3–12.9 months of age at baseline: a cluster-randomized controlled Trial. J Nutr 2015;1–8.
14 Ruel MT: Operationalizing dietary diversity: a review of measurement issues and research priorities. J Nutr 2003;133:3911S–3926S.
15 Working Group on Infant and Young Child Feeding Indicators. Developing and validating simple indicators of dietary quality and energy intake of infants and young children in developing countries: summary of findings from analysis of 10 data sets. Washington, Food and Nutrition Technical Assistance (FANTA) Project, Academy for Educational Development (AED), 2006.
16 Ruel MT, Harris J, Cunningham K: Diet quality in developing countries; in Preedy VR, Hunter L, Patel V (eds): Diet Quality. An Evidence-Based Approach, Volume 2, Nutrition and Health. New York, Springer, 2013, pp 239–261.
17 Marriott BP, White A, Hadden L, et al: World Health Organization (WHO) infant and young child feeding indicators: associations with growth measures in 14 low-income countries. Matern Child Nutr 2012;8:354–370.
18 Jones AD, Ickes SB, Smith LE, et al: World Health Organization infant and young child feeding indicators and their associations with child anthropometry: a synthesis of recent findings. Matern Child Nutr 2014;10:1–17.
19 Hall Moran V, Dewey K, Dibley MJ, Senarath U (eds): Complementary feeding practices in South Asia: Analyses by the South Asia Infant Feeding Research Network (SAIFRN). Matern Child Nutr 2012;8(suppl s1):1–106.
20 Senarath U, Agho KE, Dur-e-Samin Akram D-S, et al: Comparisons of complementary feeding indicators and associated factors in children aged 6–23 months across five South Asian countries. Matern Child Nutr 2012;8 (suppl s1):89–106.
21 Ng M, Fleming T, Robinson M, et al: Global, regional, and national prevalence of overweight and obesity in children and adults during 1980–2013: a systematic analysis for the Global Burden of Disease Study 2013. Lancet 2014;384:766–781.

Black RE, Makrides M, Ong KK (eds): Complementary Feeding: Building the Foundations for a Healthy Life. Nestlé Nutr Inst Workshop Ser, vol 87, pp 89–102, (DOI: 10.1159/000448959)
Nestec Ltd., Vevey/S. Karger AG., Basel, © 2017

Evidence for the Effects of Complementary Feeding Interventions on the Growth of Infants and Young Children in Low- and Middle-Income Countries

Rebecca A. Heidkamp
Bloomberg School of Public Health, Johns Hopkins University, Baltimore, MD, USA

Abstract
As momentum for investment in early childhood nutrition grows, so does the evidence base for the effectiveness of interventions to improve complementary feeding in low- and middle-income countries (LMIC), where the risk of early growth faltering is high. The aim of this chapter is to review the current state of the evidence for the impact of two categories of interventions (nutrition education alone and provision of food or nutrient supplements with or without education) on linear and ponderal growth of children aged 6–23 months in LMIC. Pooled-effect sizes from three recent systematic reviews consistently suggest a modest but significant effect of both types of complementary feeding interventions on weight and length gain. However, interpretation of these pooled estimates is limited by the variability in intervention design and inconsistency in reporting of growth outcomes across the relatively small number of rigorous controlled trials currently available in the literature.

Introduction

In the 2008 and 2013 *Lancet* Nutrition series, interventions to improve complementary feeding of children 6–23 months of age through caregiver education and/or provision of food supplements were cited among 10 effective nutrition interventions that, if implemented together at scale in high-burden countries, could reduce stunting by 20% and deaths in children under 5 years of age by 15% globally [1]. These projections, developed using the Lives Saved Tool, applied estimates for the effectiveness of complementary feeding interventions on growth derived from systematic reviews published around the time of the series [2–6]. As momentum for investment in early childhood nutrition interventions has grown, fueled in large part by the *Lancet* series findings, so has the evidence base for complementary feeding interventions. Given the implications for strategic planning and resource allocation by low- and middle-income country (LMIC) governments, donors, and researchers, it is important that the underlying evidence base be continuously synthesized and clearly articulated.

The aim of this chapter is to review the current state of the evidence for the impact of complementary feeding interventions on linear and ponderal growth of children aged 6–23 months in LMIC. We present findings from recent systematic reviews and select individual peer-reviewed studies. Per convention, we look separately at two broader categories of interventions: (1) education of caregivers about age-appropriate complementary feeding practices and (2) provision of foods or specially formulated supplements to complement usual intake – with or without nutrition education.

Although important for understanding how and why interventions work, examining intermediates and other outcomes along the program impact pathway from intervention to growth (e.g. changes in caregiver knowledge and practices, child dietary intake, nutrient status, morbidity, and child development) is outside the scope of this chapter.

Three systematic reviews published in the last 5 years provide pooled estimates for the growth effects of complementary feeding interventions [2, 4, 7]. Meta-analyses have recognized limitations but remain our primary tool for synthesizing evidence across intervention trials. In order to appropriately interpret and apply the resulting pooled estimates, one must clearly understand the question being addressed by the systematic review and methods used to select studies, grade quality, assess heterogeneity, and combine quantitative estimates [8]. To account for the heterogeneity in how outcomes are measured across studies, continuous outcomes may be reported as standardized mean differences (SMD) rather than absolute mean differences (MD). SMD are expressed in standard deviation units and interpreted as the relative magnitude of the effect in treatment versus control. An SMD of 0.2 is considered a small, 0.5 a medium and 0.8 a large effect [9].

Evidence for the Effect of Education-Only Interventions

Complementary feeding education interventions promote optimal caregiver practices related to continued breastfeeding, age-appropriate food choice (e.g. diversity of food groups and nutrient density), food preparation methods (e.g.

developmentally appropriate textures and food hygiene) as well as frequency and style of feeding (e.g. responsive feeding and feeding during illness) [10]. Effective behavior change communication interventions are designed and adapted for local contexts based on formative research and promote context-specific practices (e.g. consumption of specific foods that are locally accessible) [11]. Complementary feeding interventions are far more diverse than interventions such as high-dose vitamin A supplementation or even promotion of exclusive breastfeeding, where the messages and methods being promoted are fairly consistent across contexts. This diversity in design and implementation presents challenges for generating pooled effectiveness estimates [8].

A series of systematic reviews examining the impact of complementary feeding education alone on growth of children in LMIC has been published since the late 1990s [2, 5–7, 12]. The two most recent studies by Imdad et al. [7] and Lassi et al. [2] include an overlapping set of 7 intervention trials. Lassi et al. [2] identified a total of 10 trials of education-only interventions meeting inclusion criteria compared to 8 in the study by Imdad et al. [7]. Both reviews limited study inclusion to controlled intervention trials among children under 24 months in LMIC with available data on change in weight and/or length. Lassi et al. [2] further restricted their analysis to trials with a 6-month minimum intervention duration that did not selectively enroll malnourished children. Using the methods for quality assessment developed by the Child Health Epidemiology Reference Group (CHERG) [13], both reviews graded evidence for each reported growth outcome as moderate. In 2011, Imdad et al. [7] reported pooled estimates for weight and length change only, and increased the total number of studies contributing to the estimate by back calculating absolute changes in length and weight from z-scores reported in 2 studies [14, 15].

As summarized in table 1, the 2 reviews reported similar pooled estimates for relative differences in length gain and weight gain in groups receiving education-only interventions compared to no intervention controls. Imdad et al. [7] also reported absolute differences in length and weight gain, while Lassi et al. [2] reported pooled estimates for several additional growth metrics, including weight-for-age z-score (WAZ), length-for-age z-score (LAZ), and stunting. They did not report pooled estimates for weight-for-length z-score (WLZ) or wasting even though 5 of the 9 studies included in the analysis reported WLZ outcomes. The SMD in WAZ and LAZ were both small (<0.3) and not significant, but the pooled effect for stunting was larger and statistically significant [relative risk (RR) 0.71 (95% CI 0.60–0.76); 5 studies, 3 with benefit].

Lassi et al. [2] presented a subanalysis by food security status in which trials were classified as food secure or food insecure based on a country level per capita

Table 1. Effects of complementary feeding education alone on linear growth and weight gain: summary findings from recent meta-analyses

Outcomes	Imdad et al. [7], 2011			Lassi et al. [2], 2013		
	metric	pooled effect, SMD or MD (95% CI)	studies, n	population	pooled effect, SMD (95% CI)	studies, n
Height gain	relative (SMD) absolute (MD)	0.21 SD (0.01 to 0.41) 0.49 CM (–0.00 to 0.99)	7	overall food secure food insecure	0.23 SD (–0.00, 0.45) 0.35 SD (0.08, 0.62) 0.00 SD (–0.15, 0.16)	6 4 2
Weight gain	relative (SMD) absolute (MD)	0.30 SD (0.05 to 0.54) 0.30 KG (0.04, 0.55)	8	overall food secure food insecure	0.26 SD (–0.00, 0.52) 0.40 SD (0.02, 0.78) 0.06 SD (–0.13, 0.25)	7 4 3

income cutoff of USD 1.25 per day. In the subanalysis, differences in height and weight gain between intervention and control groups were only observed in food-secure populations (table 1). The same pattern did not hold for WAZ, LAZ, and stunting outcomes where, based on only 1 or 2 studies in food-insecure contexts per outcome, the magnitude of pooled effects for food-insecure contexts was equal to or larger than that for food-secure contexts. The differences in weight and height gain are consistent with the rationale that food-secure populations have more resources to implement promoted feeding practices and in turn higher potential to benefit compared to food-insecure populations. We should be cautious in interpreting this finding as meaning that food- insecure populations lack any potential to benefit from education-only interventions. Rather it appears that more studies in food-insecure settings are needed to quantify the actual effect.

Neither review attempted to pool and report effect sizes by intervention design factors such as delivery platform, intensity, age group, or duration. As shown in table 2, these characteristics varied widely among the included studies. Common delivery platforms for complementary feeding education interventions include clinic visits, community-based small groups, and/or individualized home visits. The 2016 *Lancet* Breastfeeding series included a meta-analysis of 130 breastfeeding promotion intervention trials from high-income and LMIC settings that reported the effect on breastfeeding practice by delivery platform subgroups including facility, community, and/or home [16]. We attempted to carry out a similar analysis using studies from the two meta-analyses for facility compared to home- and/or community-based complementary feeding interventions, but the total sample size was too small.

Table 2. Characteristics of select trials included in reviews: complementary feeding education alone

Characteristic	Study		
	Bhandari et al. [22], 2001	Guildan [40], 2000	Penny [41], 2005
Location	India (rural)	China (rural)	Peru (peri-urban)
Generalized food security status	Insecure	Secure	Secure
Study design and sample size	Cluster RCT I = 104 C = 104	CBA I = 250 C = 250	Cluster RCT I = 187 C = 190
Age at enrollment	4 months	Birth	Birth
Baseline nutritional status of the population	Stunting: 22% (NCHS)	Mean HAZ –0.6 (NCHS)	Mean HAZ (3 months) +0.7 (NCHS)
Delivery platform	Home visit	Home visit	Health center
Intervention design	Home visit and individualized assessment by trained community workers	Home visit with growth monitoring by trained community agents	Providers deliver 3 key messages to all children at routine visits; age-specific group education and cooking demonstration
Frequency of contact	Monthly	Monthly	9–10 visits over 18 months
Duration of exposure to intervention	8 months	12 months	18 months
Statistically significant effect on length gain?	No	Yes	Yes

C = Control; HAZ = height-for-age z-score; I = intervention; NCHS = National Center for Health Statistics.

Provision of Food or Other Supplements with or without Education

The second category of complementary feeding interventions examined in recent meta-analyses is providing food rations and/or supplements containing energy and micronutrients to children 6–23 months with or without nutrition education. In pooling outcomes of interventions with and without education together, it is assumed that the nutritional supplement drives all of the observed effect on growth. Interventions to treat severe acute malnutrition in children aged 6–23 months are not considered complementary feeding interventions as therapeutic food supplements fully displace, rather than 'complement', the usual diet. Interventions providing energy-dense lipid or cereal-based fortified food supplements to children aged 6–23 months with ‘moderate acute malnutrition’ are not as easily classified. However, most studies on moderate acute malnutrition ‘treatment’ will be excluded from complementary feeding-focused reviews based on the wider age range (6–59 months), the strategy of targeting only malnourished children, and/or differences in the time frame and outcomes reported [17].

Imdad et al. [7] and Lassi et al. [2] reported pooled effects for interventions providing food or nutrient supplements with or without education. Lassi et al. [2] identified a total of 7 trials meeting the previously described inclusion criteria compared to 11 in the study by Imdad et al. [7]. A third, more recent systematic review by Kristjansson et al. [4] examined growth outcomes of food supplementation interventions among children aged 3–59 months in LMIC. They identified 29 studies in total from LMIC that met inclusion criteria, but only 23 reported outcomes that could be used in the meta-analysis. Unlike Imdad et al. [7] and Lassi et al. [2], pooled estimates for randomized controlled trials (RCTs) and controlled before and after studies (CBA) are reported separately. Although the inclusion criteria for age applied by Kristjansson et al. [4] are broader (3–59 months) than the complementary feeding period, in 11 of the 14 RCTs from LMIC used in the meta-analysis all participants were 6–23 months. Only 2 RCTs did not include any child aged 6–23 months. Among the 9 CBAs meeting inclusion criteria for meta-analysis, 6 included participants 6–23 months of age only and none had no child in the age group. The quality of evidence for each pooled outcome across the 3 reviews was categorized as ‘moderate’ based on Grading of Recommendations, Assessments, Development and Education (GRADE)/CHERG criteria [13] except for those reported by Kristjansson et al. [4] using CBA trials which were all rated ‘very low’.

For height and weight gain, Imdad et al. [7] reported both SMD and MD which facilitate comparisons to the pooled estimates by Lassi et al. [2] using SMD and Krisjansson et al. [4] using MD. To reduce heterogeneity, Imdad et al. [7] stated findings with and without the study by Obatolu [18]. Lassi et al. [2] included the Obatolu [18] outcomes in pooled estimates.

Table 3 demonstrates the variability in intervention and study design among trials included in the reviews.

Despite the variability in the included studies, pooled effect sizes for height gain and weight gain are consistent across the 4 sets of analyses (table 4). Relative effect sizes (SMD) are small (<0.5) and significant only in the study by Imdad et al. [7]. The absolute effects on length (MD 0.43 cm, 95% CI 0.19–0.65) and weight (MD 0.14 kg, 95% CI 0.05–0.24) reported by Imdad et al. [7] (without Obatolu [18]) include both RCTs and CBAs, and fall consistently between the independent pooled estimates for RCTs (length 0.27 cm, 95% CI 0.07–0.48;

Table 3. Characteristics of select trials included in reviews: provision of food rations or energy-based nutritional supplement with or without education

Characteristics	Grantham-McGregor et al. [23], 1991	Lutter et al. [42], 2008	Mangani et al. [21], 2015	Ianotti et al. [43], 2014
Location	Jamaica (urban)	Ecuador (urban)	Malawi (rural)	Haiti (urban)
Study design and sample size	RCT I = 64; C = 33	CBA; I: 338 (170 at end) C: 296 (149 at end)	RCT; 840 total: 183–191/group × 4	RCT; C: 144 I 150 (to 3 mo) and 126 (to 6 mo)
Age at enrollment, months	19–24	9–14	6	6–11
Target malnourished kids	Yes	No	No	No
Ration type/energy content, kcal/day (% energy DRI)	Milk based/750 (9–12 mo 105%; 12–24 mo 86.3%]	Milk based/275 [9–12 mo 38.6%; 12–24 mo 31.6%]	LNS or CSB/ 276–284 (~40%)	LNS/108 (15%)
Duration of exposure to the intervention, mo	24	11	12	6
Statistically significant effect on length gain?	Yes during first 6 mo (younger)	No	No	Yes

C = Control; CSB = corn soy blend; I = intervention; mo = months; DRI = dietary reference intake.

weight 0.12 kg, 95% CI 0.05–0.18) and CBAs (length 0.52 cm, 95% CI –0.07 to 1.1; weight 0.24 kg, 95% CI 0.09–0.39) reported by Kristjansson et al. [4]. A similar pattern is seen when comparing WAZ and LAZ, with the exception of the nonsignificant effect on LAZ in the CBA analysis by Kristjansson et al. [4]. Only Lassi et al. [2] reported significant pooled effects on underweight (RR 0.35, 95% CI 0.16–0.77; 1 study) and stunting (RR 0.33, 95% CI 0.11–1.00; 7 studies, 2 with benefit). Pooled effects on weight-for-height z-scores were not significant for RCTs or CBAs in Krisjansson et al. [4], the only meta-analysis to report this outcome.

All studies pooled by Lassi et al. [2] for this intervention category were from countries classified as food insecure. The authors recommend that pooled effect sizes be generalized only to similar food-insecure populations.

Kristjansson et al. [4] carried out a series of subgroup analyses relevant to intervention design and delivery factors, including classifying studies by nutrient adequacy of the supplement (examples in table 3). Among the RCTs, the effects of interventions providing high-energy supplements (>60% DRI) on height compared to control were large and statically significant (MD 0.62 cm, 95% CI 0.13–1.11; 2 studies) in comparison to those providing medium (30–59% DRI)

Table 4. Effects of complementary feeding interventions providing food or nutrition supplements on linear growth and weight gain: summary of findings from three recent meta-analysis

Outcome	Imdad et al. [7], 2011			Lassi et al. [2], 2013			Kristjansson et al. [4], 2015 – RCT			Kristjansson et al. [4], 2015 – CBA		
	pooled effect SMD/MD (95% CI)	total sample size	studies, n	pooled effect SMD (95% CI)	total sample size	studies, n	pooled effect MD (95% CI)	total sample size	studies, n	pooled effect MD (95% CI)	total sample size	studies, n
Height gain	With Obatolu [18], 2003: SMD 0.26 SD (0.08–0.43), MD 0.54 cm (0.16–0.9) Without Obatolu: SMD 0.19 (0.04–0.33) MD 0.43 cm (0.19–0.65)	n.r.	11 total (SMD 4, MD 4)	0.34 SD (–0.09, 0.78)	512	4 (2)	0.27 cm (0.07, 0.48)	1,463	9	0.52 cm (–0.07, 1.1)	1,782	7 (n.a.)
Weight gain	With Obatolu: SMD 0.34 SD (0.11–0.56) MD 0.25 kg (0.07–0.44) Without Obatolu: SMD 0.22 SD (0.06–0.38) MD 0.14 kg (0.05–0.24)	n.r.	11 total (SMD 4, MD 6)	0.43 SD (–0.42, 1.27)	512	4 (1)	0.12 kg (0.05, 0.18)	1,057	9 (n.r.)	0.24 kg (0.09, 0.39)	1,784	7 (n.a.)
ΔWAZ	–	–	–	0.26 SD (0.04, 0.48)	318	3 (1)	0.15 SD (0.05, 0.24)	1,565	8 (n.r.)	0.27 SD (0.1, 0.68)	999	4 (n.r.)
ΔLAZ	–	–	–	0.39 SD (0.05, 0.73)	1,652	7 (2)	0.15 SD (0.06, 0.24)	4,544	9 (n.r.)	0.01 SD (–0.10,0.12)	999	4 (n.r.)
ΔWLZ	–	–	–	–	–	–	0.10 SD (–0.02, 0.22)	4,073	6 (n.r.)	0.29 SD (–0.11, 0.69)	999	4 (n.r.)

(MD 0.16 cm, 95% CI –0.09 to 0.41; 5 studies) or low energy (0–29% DRI) supplements (MD 0.25 cm, 95% CI –0.05 to 0.55; 1 study). There were no statistically significant differences in weight gain across subgroups. Kristjansson et al. [4] did not consider the type of supplement (e.g. milk-based, corn soy blend, or lipid-based nutrient supplements, LNS) in their analyses, but several individual RCTs comparing various formulations of LNS (e.g. locally produced, milk-based, soy-based LNS) to fortified cereals or flours with similar energy and micronutrient composition do not report significant differences in absolute length or weight gain by supplement type [19–21].

Consistent with findings reported in much earlier reviews [5], additional subanalyses presented by Kristjansson et al. [4] suggested trends towards improved growth outcomes for younger or more malnourished children, for interventions involving center-based compared to home-based feeding, and for multifaceted interventions (e.g. supplementation with stimulation) compared to single strategy interventions (e.g. supplementation alone). Small sample sizes limit the ability to draw conclusions. In an exploratory analysis, Kristjansson et al. [4] pooled effects from 3 RCTs [22–24] they characterized as being particularly well implemented based on factors including sufficiency of ration, adherence, and supervision. The pooled estimate for height gain (0.76 cm, 95% CI 0.30–1.22; intervention: n = 137 and control: n = 144) from these 3 was much higher than that reported for all studies in table 4.

Two trials included in one or more of the systematic reviews used supplements that qualify as *small-quantity lipid-based nutrient supplements (SQ-LNS),* a new form of multiple micronutrient supplements designed for the complementary feeding age group. SQ-LNS contain a complete daily requirement of micronutrients for children aged 6–23 months in about 20 g of a lipid-based matrix that provides <120 kcal energy, some protein, and essential fatty acids. A 2007 RCT in Ghana (included in Lassi et al. [2] and Imdad et al. [7]) among children aged 6–12 months was the first trial testing the effects of SQ-LNS on growth and reported a small nonsignificant effect on linear growth [25]. More recently, an RCT in an urban slum of Haiti [26] (included in Kristjansson et al. [4]) provided SQ-LNS daily for 3 or 6 months to children aged 6–11 months at baseline. They reported high compliance and a greater age-adjusted increase in LAZ (mean ± SE) 0.13 ± 0.05 and WAZ 0.12 ± 0.02 after 6 months (n = 202) compared to control (n = 191; p = 0.001). Two additional RCTs testing SQ-LNS have been published since 2015 and report mixed results. A cluster RCT in rural Burkina Faso [27] (baseline stunting 20–23%) testing SQ-LNS formulations with variable doses of zinc found children receiving any SQ-LNS type from age 9 to 18 months (n = 2,435) were longer at 18 months compared to the no intervention controls (n = 785) (77.7 ± 3.0 vs. 76.9 ± 3.4cm; p < 0.001). Prevalence of stunting (29.3 vs.

39.3%; $p < 0.0001$) and wasting (8.7 vs. 13.5%; $p = 0.0003$) also decreased. In contrast, an RCT in rural Malawi [28] assigned women to one of three different supplements during pregnancy through 6 months postpartum (iron, folic acid, multiple micronutrient tablets, and SQ-LNS) and then provided SQ-LNS to offspring of the SQ-LNS prenatal supplementation from 6 to 18 months of age. There were no differences in growth outcomes between child groups at 18 months in unadjusted or adjusted analyses, and overall prevalence of stunting at the last follow-up was very high (32.7–37.9%). Generally, SQ-LNS appears to have potential for small effects on growth in LMIC. Growth effects at 18 months should be forthcoming from at least one other pre- and postnatal trial in Ghana [29], and once available, a pooled analysis of these SQ-LNS studies using standardized outcomes is called for.

Although they do not contain energy (and therefore were not considered in any of the three systematic reviews discussed above), *multiple micronutrient powders* (MNP) are another form of multiple micronutrient supplement recommended by the WHO for home-based fortification of complementary foods in populations with high anemia burden. Individual MNP sachets contain a recommended daily intake of two or more problem nutrients for the targeted age group and generally include zinc. A 2013 review of 17 studies concluded that although MNP have an impact on iron status and anemia in children aged 6–59 months, none of the 3 studies (4 datasets) reporting anthropometric outcomes showed an impact on growth [30]. Beyond implementation issues including adherence, the lack of growth effects across these trials may be explained in part by the relatively lower dose of zinc in MNP compared to zinc-only supplements in trials [31, 32], a reduction in zinc bioavailability due to high phytic acid content of foods mixed with the MNP, and the adverse effects of iron supplements on diarrhea and growth [33, 34].

Characterizing the Overall Evidence Base

Evidence from meta-analyses of controlled trials consistently points to the potential for complementary feeding interventions to have a modest but significant impact on growth of children aged 6–23 months in LMIC. However, at present, there is not sufficient evidence based on the number and variety of large-scale trials to support meaningful categorization and comparison of growth effects across subtypes of interventions that would be meaningful to policy makers and program planners based on population (e.g. child age or baseline nutritional status), design (e.g. delivery platform for education interventions), and/or delivery (e.g. duration or intensity of supervision) factors.

There are few examples of complementary feeding intervention effectiveness evaluations that have been purposefully designed to facilitate pooled effect estimates and/or cross-context comparisons. An evaluation study in Pakistan [35] of the facility-based nutrition counseling component of the Integrated Management for Childhood Illness strategy replicated the approach of an earlier trial in Brazil [36]. More recently, in addition to the SQ-LNS trials presented earlier, coordinated trials have been carried out in Guatemala and Burundi to test the 'PM2A' strategy for targeting food supplements that was first evaluated in rural Haiti [37].

Even though complementary feeding intervention trials consistently collect height and weight data, our ability to pool results of trials is further limited by inconsistencies in which outcomes are reported. This likely stems in part from changes over time in which outcomes are of greatest interest to the research and practice communities as well as recognized biases to statistically significant positive results. Early studies from the 1980s to 1990s, primarily reported changes in weight-related indicators. Over the last 10 years, interventions have been evaluated with linear growth as the priority outcome [2]. Currently, there is growing interest in the potential for complementary feeding interventions to prevent wasting, but many studies have not systematically reported outcomes of weight-for-height z-scores or wasting.

Fortunately, the overall quality of trials has improved over time [4] and guidance is available to facilitate more consistent and complete reporting of complex intervention designs and results [38, 39]. To facilitate cross-study analyses, authors should use web annexes to consistently report all growth outcomes based on weight and height measures (e.g. absolute change, z-score, %<-2SD) in the intervention and comparison arms and by age subgroups whenever feasible.

Conclusion

With current efforts to scale up early childhood nutrition policies and programs globally, we are optimistic that the evidence base for growth effects of complementary feeding education interventions will continue to expand. The aim is to characterize differences across meaningful typologies of complementary feeding interventions based on both design and population factors.

Disclosure Statement

The author has no conflicts of interest to report.

References

1 Bhutta ZA, Das JK, Rizvi A, et al: Evidence-based interventions for improvement of maternal and child nutrition: what can be done and at what cost? Lancet 2013;382:452–477.

2 Lassi ZS, Das JK, Zahid G, et al: Impact of education and provision of complementary feeding on growth and morbidity in children less than 2 years of age in developing countries: a systematic review. BMC Public Health 2013;13:1–10.

3 Lassi ZS, Das JK, Zahid G, et al: Impact of education and provision of complementary feeding on growth and morbidity in children less than 2 years of age in developing countries: a systematic review. BMC Public Health 2013;13(suppl 3):S13.

4 Kristjansson E, Francis DK, Liberato S, et al: Food supplementation for improving the physical and psychosocial health of socio-economically disadvantaged children aged three months to five years. Cochrane Database Syst Rev 2015;3:CD009924.

5 Dewey KG, Adu-Afarwuah S: Systematic review of the efficacy and effectiveness of complementary feeding interventions in developing countries. Matern Child Nutr 2008; 4(suppl 1):24–85.

6 Bhutta ZA, Ahmed T, Black RE, et al: What works? Interventions for maternal and child undernutrition and survival. Lancet 2008; 371:417–440.

7 Imdad A, Yakoob MY, Bhutta ZA: Impact of maternal education about complementary feeding and provision of complementary foods on child growth in developing countries. BMC Public Health 2011;11(suppl 3):S25.

8 Ioannidis JP, Lau J: Pooling research results: benefits and limitations of meta-analysis. Jt Comm J Qual Improv 1999;25:462–469.

9 Cohen J: Statistical Power Analysis for the Behavioral Sciences. Hillsdale, Erlbaum, 1988.

10 Pan American Health Organization (PAHO): Guiding principles for complementary feeding of the breastfed child. Geneva, WHO, 2003, http://www.who.int/maternal_child_adolescent/documents/a85622/en/.

11 Fabrizio CS, van Liere M, Pelto G: Identifying determinants of effective complementary feeding behaviour change interventions in developing countries. Matern Child Nutr 2014;10:575–592.

12 Caulfield LE, Huffman SL: Interventions to Improve Intake of Complementary Foods by Infants 6 to 12 Months of Age in Developing Countries: Impact on Growth and on the Prevalence of Malnutrition and Potential Contribution to Child Survival. Food Nutr Bull 1999, https://www.researchgate.net/publication/243783715_Interventions_to_Improve_Intake_of_Complementary_Foods_by_Infants_6_to_12_Months_of_Age_in_Developing_Countries_Impact_on_Growth_and_on_the_Prevalence_of_Malnutrition_and_Potential_Contribution_to_Chi.

13 Walker N, Fischer-Walker C, Bryce J, et al, CHERG Review Groups on Intervention Effects: Standards for CHERG reviews of intervention effects on child survival. Int J Epidemiol 2010;39(suppl. 1):i21–i31.

14 Guldan GS, Fan HC, Ma X, et al: Culturally appropriate nutrition education improves infant feeding and growth in rural Sichuan, China. J Nutr 2000;130:1204–1211.

15 Roy SK, Fuchs GJ, Mahmud Z, et al: Intensive nutrition education with or without supplementary feeding improves the nutritional status of moderately malnourished children in Bangladesh. J Health Popul Nutr 2005;23: 320–330.

16 Sinha B, Chowdhury R, Sankar MJ, et al: Interventions to improve breastfeeding outcomes: a systematic review and meta-analysis. Acta Paediatr 2015;104:114–134.

17 Lazzerini M, Rubert L, Pani P: Specially formulated foods for treating children with moderate acute malnutrition in low- and middle-income countries. Cochrane Database Syst Rev 2013;6:CD009584.

18 Obatolu VA: Growth pattern of infants fed with a mixture of extruded malted maize and cowpea. Nutrition 2003;19:174–178.

19 Christian P, Shaikh S, Shamim AA, et al: Effect of fortified complementary food supplementation on child growth in rural Bangladesh: a cluster-randomized trial. Int J Epidemiol 2015;44:1862–1876.

20 Phuka J, Thakwalakwa C, Maleta K, et al: Supplementary feeding with fortified spread among moderately underweight 6- to 18-month-old rural Malawian children. Matern Child Nutr 2009;5:159–170.

21 Mangani C, Maleta K, Phuka J, et al: Effect of complementary feeding with lipid-based nutrient supplements and corn-soy blend on the incidence of stunting and linear growth among 6- to 18-month-old infants and children in rural Malawi. Matern Child Nutr 2015;11(suppl 4):132–143.
22 Bhandari N, Bahl R, Nayyar B, et al: Food supplementation with encouragement to feed it to infants from 4 to 12 months of age has a small impact on weight gain. J Nutr 2001;131: 1946–1951.
23 Grantham-McGregor SM, Powell CA, Walker SP, et al: Nutritional supplementation, psychosocial stimulation, and mental development of stunted children: the Jamaican Study. Lancet 1991;338:1–5.
24 Kuusipalo H, Maleta K, Briend A, et al: Growth and change in blood haemoglobin concentration among underweight Malawian infants receiving fortified spreads for 12 weeks: a preliminary trial. J Pediatr Gastroenterol Nutr 2006;43:525–532.
25 Adu-Afarwuah S, Lartey A, Brown KH, et al: Randomized comparison of 3 types of micronutrient supplements for home fortification of complementary foods in Ghana: effects on growth and motor development. Am J Clin Nutr 2007;86:412–420.
26 Iannotti LL, Dulience SJL, Green J, et al: Linear growth increased in young children in an urban slum of Haiti: a randomized controlled trial of a lipid-based nutrient supplement. Am J Clin Nutr 2014;99:198–208.
27 Hess SY, Abbeddou S, Jimenez EY, et al: Small-quantity lipid-based nutrient supplements, regardless of their zinc content, increase growth and reduce the prevalence of stunting and wasting in young Burkinabe children: a cluster-randomized trial. PLoS One 2015;10:e0122242.
28 Ashorn P, Alho L, Ashorn U, et al: The impact of lipid-based nutrient supplement provision to pregnant women on newborn size in rural Malawi: a randomized controlled trial. Am J Clin Nutr 2015;101:387–397.
29 Adu-Afarwuah S, Lartey A, Okronipa H, et al: Lipid-based nutrient supplement increases the birth size of infants of primiparous women in Ghana. Am J Clin Nutr 2015;101:835–846.
30 Salam RA, MacPhail C, Das JK, et al: Effectiveness of micronutrient powders (MNP) in women and children. BMC Public Health 2013;13(suppl 3):S22.
31 Soofi S, Cousens S, Iqbal SP, et al: Effect of provision of daily zinc and iron with several micronutrients on growth and morbidity among young children in Pakistan: a cluster-randomised trial. Lancet 2013;382:29–40.
32 De-Regil LM, Suchdev PS, Vist GE, et al: Home fortification of foods with multiple micronutrient powders for health and nutrition in children under two years of age. Cochrane Database Syst Rev 2011;9: CD008959.
33 Gera T, Sachdev HPS: Effect of iron supplementation on incidence of infectious illness in children: systematic review. BMJ 2002;325: 1142.
34 Dewey KG, Domellöf M, Cohen RJ, et al: Iron supplementation affects growth and morbidity of breast-fed infants: results of a randomized trial in Sweden and Honduras. J Nutr 2002;132:3249–3255.
35 Zaman S, Ashraf RN, Martines J: Training in complementary feeding counselling of healthcare workers and its influence on maternal behaviours and child growth: a cluster-randomized controlled trial in Lahore, Pakistan. J Health Popul Nutr 2008;26: 210–222.
36 Santos I, Victora CG, Martines J, et al: Nutrition counseling increases weight gain among Brazilian children. J Nutr 2001;131:2866–2873.
37 Ruel MT, Menon P, Habicht J-P, et al: Age-based preventive targeting of food assistance and behaviour change and communication for reduction of childhood undernutrition in Haiti: a cluster randomised trial. Lancet 2008; 371:588–595.
38 Möhler R, Bartoszek G, Meyer G: Quality of reporting of complex healthcare interventions and applicability of the CReDECI list – a survey of publications indexed in PubMed. BMC Med Res Methodol 2013;13:125.
39 Armstrong R, Waters E, Moore L, et al: Improving the reporting of public health intervention research: advancing TREND and CONSORT. J Public Health (Oxf) 2008;30: 103–109.

40 Guldan GS, Fan HC, Ma X, et al: Culturally appropriate nutrition education improves infant feeding and growth in rural Sichuan, China. J Nutr 2000;130:1204–1211.
41 Penny ME, Creed-Kanashiro HM, Robert RC, et al: Effectiveness of an educational intervention delivered through the health services to improve nutrition in young children: a cluster-randomised controlled trial. Lancet 2005;365:1863–1872.
42 Lutter CK, Rodríguez A, Fuenmayor G, et al: Growth and micronutrient status in children receiving a fortified complementary food. J Nutr 2008;138:379–388.
43 Iannotti LL, Dulience SJ, Green J, et al: Linear growth increased in young children in an urban slum of Haiti: a randomized controlled trial of a lipid-based nutrient supplement. Am J Clin Nutr 2014;99:198–208.

Black RE, Makrides M, Ong KK (eds): Complementary Feeding: Building the Foundations for a Healthy Life. Nestlé Nutr Inst Workshop Ser, vol 87, pp 103–113, (DOI: 10.1159/000448960)
Nestec Ltd., Vevey/S. Karger AG., Basel, © 2017

Results with Complementary Food Using Local Food Ingredients

Tahmeed Ahmed · Munirul Islam · Nuzhat Choudhury · Iqbal Hossain · Sayeeda Huq · Mustafa Mahfuz · Shafiqul Alam Sarker

Nutrition and Clinical Services Division, icddr,b, Dhaka, Bangladesh

Abstract

Appropriate complementary food is a must for optimum growth of infants and children. The food should be diverse and be given in sufficient quantities 2–4 times a day depending upon age. Poverty, food insecurity, and lack of awareness regarding the choice of nutritious food ingredients are deterrents to optimum complementary feeding. In Bangladesh, 77% of children do not receive appropriate complementary food and, hence, the high prevalence of childhood malnutrition. We developed ready-to-use complementary foods (RUCFs) using locally available food ingredients, rice/lentil and chickpea, which conform to standard specifications. These foods were found to be acceptable by children and their mothers compared to the Pushti packet, the cereal-based supplement used in the erstwhile National Nutrition Program of Bangladesh. In a cluster-randomized community-based trial in rural Bangladesh among more than 5,000 children, the efficacy of rice/lentil- and chickpea-based RUCFs was compared with another commonly used supplementary food called wheat-soy blend++ (WSB++) and a commercial product called Plumpy'doz. Deceleration in length for age was significantly lower (by 0.02–0.04/month) in the rice/lentil, Plumpy'doz, and chickpea groups compared to the control group at 18 months of age. Weight-for-length z-score decline was lower only in Plumpy'doz and chickpea groups. WSB++ was not different from the control group. In children who received chickpea RUCF or Plumpy'doz, the prevalence of stunting was 5–6% lower at 18 months. These foods can be used to prevent or treat malnutrition among children, particularly those from food-insecure households.

Introduction

Up to 6 months, an infant should be fed only mother's breast milk. After the first 6 months, breast milk alone is not enough, and complementary food should be given in addition to breast milk up to at least 2 years. When the child is 6 months old, the supply of energy and iron, among other nutrients, may be limited in breast milk, which can then supply only 60–70 and 6–7% of the required intakes of energy and iron, respectively [1]. Existing Infant and Young Child Feeding (IYCF) guidelines provide a robust guidance on complementary feeding of infants and young children. IYCF guidelines categorize food for children into seven groups, which include: (1) grains, roots, and tubers; (2) legumes and nuts; (3) milk, yogurt, and cheese; (4) meat and fish; (5) eggs; (6) vitamin A-rich fruits and vegetables, and (7) other fruits and vegetables [2]. It is recommended that children after 6 months of age daily take food from at least four food groups, in order not to become nutrient deficient (minimum dietary diversity). The MAD (minimally accepted diet) is an important metric for assessing quality of complementary food for children. It is a composite of taking food from at least four of the above-mentioned food groups including milk and a daily feeding frequency of 2–4 times depending on age. In Bangladesh, only 23% of children under 2 years receive MAD [2]. These figures are 26.5 and 5.8% for Nepal and Uganda, respectively [3, 4].

Children receive inappropriate complementary diets for various reasons, which include poverty, food insecurity, and lack of awareness regarding appropriate child feeding practices. Poverty and food insecurity are inseparable. The projected reduction in poverty based on the upper poverty line cost of basic needs is 24.8% in 2015 compared to 29.9% in 2011. Extreme poverty, on the other hand, as defined as head count below the lower poverty line is projected to be reduced marginally from 16.5% in 2011 to 12.9% in 2015 [5]. Food insecurity, assessed on the basis of consumption of <1,805 kcal per capita per day, affects 16% of the Bangladeshi population [6]. In a study done in rural Bangladesh, we assessed the adequacy of intake of 11 micronutrients among 24- to 48-month-old children. The overall mean prevalence of adequacy of micronutrient intake for children was only 43%. The prevalence of adequacy was less than 50% for iron, calcium, riboflavin, folate, and vitamin B_{12} [7]. This inadequacy of the micronutrient status among children in Bangladesh was explained by the intake of diets low in energy and little diversity of foods. In the same study, we observed that almost all women consumed less than the recommended intake levels for total fat, total polyunsaturated fatty acids, α-linolenic acid (ALA) and docosahexaenoic acid. Median breast milk linoleic acid (8.5% of weight) and ALA (0.2%) concentrations were among the lowest reported in the literature. We also observed that children consumed suboptimal amounts of fat, and in most children only 1–4% of the total energy came from essential fatty acids [8]. More than 95% of the children had fat intakes <30% of total energy. An estimated 80% of all the children consumed <4% of total energy as linoleic acid, and 99% consumed <1% of energy as ALA, implying an acute lack of essential fatty acids in the diet.

It is, therefore, clear that poor essential fatty acid concentrations in the breast milk and MAD contribute to the huge burden of childhood malnutrition in Bangladesh. With an annual 1.4% reduction in the prevalence of linear growth retardation or stunting (length-for-age z-score, LAZ, <–2 SD), 36% of children below 5 years still suffer from stunting. Given the current pace, it will be a challenge to achieve the World Health Assembly target of reducing stunting by 40% by 2025 [9]. There has been little improvement in acute malnutrition or wasting (weight-for-length z-score, WLZ, <–2 SD), and currently 14% of children below 5 years suffer from this condition. Many of these children slide into the deadly form of malnutrition called severe acute malnutrition or severe wasting (WLZ <–2 SD or a mid-upper arm circumference <115 mm or bilateral pedal edema). In Bangladesh, the current prevalence of severe acute malnutrition is 3%, which implies about 450,000 children. Underweight (weight for age z-score, WAZ, <–2 SD) affects 33% children.

The Need for Improved Complementary Food

The preparation of complementary food at home with the use of the food ingredients from the IYCF food groups is ideal and should be promoted. But this is not always possible for families that are poor and food insecure. People who live in hard-to-reach areas are vulnerable to severe food insecurity, e.g., people living in temporary shelters built on river shoals that are subject to river erosion and those who subsist on social safety net programs. There is, therefore, a need to top up diet of such children with adequate energy, fat, and protein, including animal source protein. This is more applicable for children with moderate acute malnutrition for whom a WHO convening has recommended 25 kcal per kilogram body weight in addition to what is required for healthy peers and the inclusion of animal source food in the diet [10]. Under dire conditions of inadequate water, sanitation, and hygiene practices, which are prevalent in many communities in developing countries, it is not always possible to prepare and store complementary food at home free of microbial contamination. In a study in villages and an urban slum in Bangladesh, we investigated the microbiological quality of complementary foods and its association with diarrheal morbidity and nutritional status [11]. Around 40% of complementary food samples were contaminated with *Escherichia coli*, which was mainly attributable to faulty food preparation. Consumption of contaminated complementary food was associated with a higher frequency of diarrhea and malnutrition in children.

Development of Improved Complementary Food Using Local Food Ingredients

Since inadequate energy and micronutrient intake during childhood is a major public health problem in developing countries which are plagued with food insecurity, we developed ready-to-use complementary food (RUCF) made of locally available food ingredients [12]. This was designed to have the required amount of micronutrients essential for growth and development of children 6–24 months of age. RUCF does not require cooking and can be consumed without adding water either on its own or by mixing with other food such as rice porridge. It has minimal water content and, thus, the risk of contamination or bacterial growth is greatly reduced. These characteristics make provision of RUCF a safe nutrition for young children in Bangladesh. We did a yearlong market survey to look at the availability and stability of prices of local food ingredients. Three ingredients were selected: rice, lentils, and chickpea. The theoretical formulation of RUCF components was made based on linear programming to identify the combinations of ingredients and micronutrient premixes that would result in the most nutritious recipes. Linear programming is based on a mathematical iterative approach involving multiple calculations of products and sums that can be quickly performed by a personal computer. Two recipes were prepared: one based on rice/lentil and the other on chickpea. The total energy obtained from 50 g of rice/lentil- and chickpea-based RUCFs were 264 and 267 kcal, respectively, which also supplied ~70% of the micronutrient needs of a child (table 1). The experiments for developing RUCFs and assessing the shelf life were performed in the Food Processing Laboratory of icddr,b. We produced the recipes in small batches by mixing all ingredients in an electric blender. When necessary, consistency of the recipe was adjusted by varying the amount of dry ingredients and soybean oil. The combination of minerals and vitamins were adjusted to avoid an unpleasant taste, which can occur with the addition of a high dose of micronutrients. We added a small amount (1%) of soy lecithin to the recipe to improve the consistency and prevent oil separation. During the development stage, microbiological tests (total viable count, yeasts, molds, coliforms, *E. coli*, *Bacillus cereus,* staphylococci, *Listeria monocytogenes*, and *Cronobacter sakazakii*) were performed at the icddr,b Food Safety Laboratory. Chemical properties (pH, water activity, moisture, peroxide value, and total aflatoxin),

Table 1. Composition of RUCF and the Pushti packet per serving of 50 g

	Rice-lentil-based RUCF	Chickpea-based RUCF	Pushti packet
Energy, kcal	264	267	188
Moisture, g	1.0	1.2	n.d.
Protein, g	5.1	6	4.9
Total fat, g	14.8	15.9	4.2
Carbohydrates, g	27.6	24.9	32.6
Dietary fiber, g	1.1	0.6	n.d.
Ash, g	1.95	2.5	n.d.
Vitamin A, μg	427.5	294	0.39
β-Carotene, μg	8.5	26.5	n.d.
Vitamin C, mg	16	20.5	0.65
Vitamin E, mg	10.41	14.0	n.d.
Vitamin B_1 mg	0.475	0.78	0.07
Vitamin B_2, mg	0.515	0.63	0.04
Calcium, mg	286.0	413.3	0
Phosphorus, mg	240	318	n.d.
Sodium, mg	20.5	37	n.d.
Potassium, mg	317	424.5	n.d.
Magnesium, mg	51.425	71.5	n.d.
Iron, mg	5.905	7.0	1.92
Copper, mg	0.34	0.4	n.d.
Zinc, mg	4.15	4.9	0.80
Chloride, mg	38.5	68.5	n.d.
Aflatoxin	Not detected	Not detected	n.d.
Water activity, 24.6°C	0.32	0.32	n.d.
pH	6.3	4.1	n.d.
Peroxide value	0.2	0	n.d.

n.d. = Not determined.

nutritional composition (protein, fat, energy, and carbohydrates), and micronutrient composition were determined at the Institute of Nutrition, Mahidol University, Thailand.

Acceptability of Ready-to-Use Complementary Food Made of Locally Available Food Ingredients

We carried out an open-label acceptability trial among 6- to 18-month-old children living in an underprivileged slum community in Mirpur, Dhaka. The primary outcome variable for the acceptability trial was to see the acceptability of RUCF or the Pushti packet by measuring the amount of food consumed by children. The Pushti packet is a cereal-based food supplement used in the erstwhile National Nutrition Program of Bangladesh (table 1). The secondary outcome variable was to measure children's mothers' opinion on the food color, flavor, mouth feel, and overall acceptability by using a seven-point hedonic scale. We hypothesized that the mean consumption of RUCFs during the acceptability trial would be at least 40% of the amount offered. Assuming a standard deviation of consumption to be 15% of the amount offered, a sample size of 30 for each diet would, therefore, allow us to reject the null hypothesis with 80% power if the true means were at least 60%. The sample size was also adjusted for multiple comparisons using the Bonferroni correction. Children did not meet the enrollment criteria if their WAZ or WLZ was <–3, or if they had any acute illness or features suggestive of any chronic disease (such as tuberculosis) or congenital anomalies (such as trisomy 21, cleft lip, or palate).

Of 135 children identified from 6,152 households, 90 children were assigned to three study groups (rice/lentil- or chickpea-based RUCF, or the Pushti packet) using simple random sampling. Since the Pushti packet does not contain any added micronutrients, we gave 1 sachet of Pushtikona (Renata Limited, Dhaka), which is a micronutrient powder containing 15 micronutrients (vitamin A 0.4 mg, vitamin C 30 mg, vitamin D 0.005 mg, vitamin E 5 mg, thiamine 0.5 mg, riboflavin 0.5 mg, niacin 6 mg, pyridoxine 0.5 mg, cyanocobalamin 0.0009 mg, folic acid 0.15 mg, iron 10 mg, zinc 4.1 mg, copper 0.56 mg, selenium 0.017 mg, and iodine 0.09 mg).

The total energy obtained from 50 g of rice/lentil- and chickpea-based RUCFs and the Pushti packet were 264, 267, and 188 kcal, respectively. Children were offered 50 g of RUCF and they consumed (mean ± SD) 23.8 ± 14 g rice/lentil-based RUCF or 28.4 ± 15 g chickpea-based RUCF. The Pushti packet was also offered (50 g), but mothers were allowed to add water, and children consumed 17.1 ± 14 g.

Mean feeding time for two RUCFs and the Pushti packet was 20.9 min. Although the two RUCFs did not differ in the amount consumed, there was a significant difference in consumption between chickpea-based RUCF and the Pushti packet ($p = 0.012$) (table 2). On the 7-point hedonic scale, mean response for each sensory quality (color, flavor, mouth feel, and overall liking by mother's opinion) of all foods was more than 6. The rice/lentil- and chickpea-based RUCFs were significantly better than the Pushti packet in terms of 'overall liking'.

Efficacy of Ready-to-Use Complementary Food Made of Locally Available Food Ingredients

We tested the efficacy of the local RUCFs by an unblinded cluster-randomized controlled trial in rural Bangladesh where the effect of the two local RUCFs and a fortified blended food (wheat-soy blend++, WSB++) was compared with a

Table 2. Results of test feeding of RUCF

	Rice/ lentil-based RUCF (1)	Chickpea-based RUCF (2)	Pushti packet (3)	p value ANOVA	p value (post hoc)		
					1 vs. 2	2 vs. 3	1 vs. 3
Mean hedonic scale (mean ± SD)							
Color of the supplement	6.9±0.2	6.9±0.3	6.8±0.4	n.s.	–	–	–
Aroma/flavor of the supplement	6.8±.04	6.8±0.3	6.5±0.6	0.042	n.s.	0.049	ns
Texture/mouth feel	6.7±0.4	6.8±0.3	6.2±0.7	0.000	n.s.	0.000	0.002
Overall liking	6.9±0.2	6.9±0.3	6.4±0.6	0.000	n.s.	0.000	0.000
Amount offered, g	50.4±0.5	50.2±0.5	49.9±1.2	n.s.	–	–	–
After adding water			118.0±12				
Amount consumed, g	23.8±14	28.4±15	17.1±1	0.015	n.s.	0.012	n.s.
After adding water			40.8±35				
Food taken from offered food, %	47.2±28	56.7±31	34.4±28	0.017	n.s.	0.014	n.s.
Energy received from consumed food, kcal	125±76	152±83	64±53	0.000	n.s.	0.000	0.005
Feeding time, min	23.0±10	20.7±10	20.4±7	n.s.	–	–	–
Velocity, g/min	1.3±1.0	1.9±2.2	0.8±0.8	0.020	n.s.	0.016	n.s.

n.s. = Nonsignificant at the 5% level.

commercial lipid-based nutritional supplement called Plumpy'doz (the 'standard'), all with nutrition counseling versus nutrition counseling alone (control) [13]. The trial was done in rural communities of north western Bangladesh under the JiVitA Project of the Johns Hopkins University.

The hypothesis was that compared with nutrition counseling alone (control), each of the four complementary food products given daily for 12 months in addition to nutrition counseling would increase LAZ and WLZ by >0.2 z-scores, improve linear growth, and reduce the prevalence rates of stunting (by 10% or more) and wasting at 18 months. Additionally, each of the three complementary food products would be as good as the lipid-based Plumpy'doz for an effect on growth, with an inferiority margin of 0.2 z-scores at 18 months of age. Sample size was estimated for a noninferiority cluster-randomized trial. Available data and assumptions for the sample size estimate included the following: an endpoint LAZ in the control group of –1.70 with a standard deviation of 1.0, a mean difference in endpoint LAZ or WLZ of up to 0.2 between the three complementary food products and the standard, power 90%, type 2 error 0.05, and an attrition rate of 5%. Since the three intervention arms were compared with each of the control and standard groups, the size of the comparison groups was multiplied by a correction factor of 1.7 (the square root of the number of intervention groups, n = 3). This resulted in a final sample size of 831 children per intervention group and 1,413 children in the control and standard groups, for a total of 5,319 (rounded to 5,320) children.

The 596 predefined communities in JiVitA, called 'sectors', were cluster randomized by blocks of 19 (total 32 blocks; the last block had 7 sectors). A block number was assigned to each sector in groups of 19. For blocks 1–31, the first 5 sectors were assigned to treatment group 1, the next 5 to treatment group 2, and so on. For block 32, the two larger controls were assigned 2 sectors and the three intervention groups 1 sector each. This resulted in 157 sectors assigned to each of the control groups and 94 sectors assigned to each of the intervention groups.

Each sector was assigned to a field distributor (FD) who visited the homes of enrolled children to provide the foods and to assess daily morbidity. The FDs visited the homes twice each week to count sachets and ask about daily consumption of the complementary food. Maternal recall at each visit was used to obtain daily histories of the amount of complementary food offered to and consumed by the child. During the twice-weekly home visits, FDs also obtained a daily history of fever, cough, difficulty/rapid breathing, diarrhea, and dysentery. A weekly supply of 7 (or 14 for older children) sachets was provided once every week. Complementary foods were isocaloric and given daily at doses of 250 kcal/day. Half the dose (125 kcal) was given to infants 6–12 months of age. Plumpy'doz was provided in light-protected, lidded plastic pots of 325 g, with one pot intended to be consumed every 2 weeks at the younger age (~23 g or 1.5 table spoons/day). WSB++ was procured in 1.5-kg packs, repackaged into daily portions of 32 g of flour, and delivered at home to be cooked into a water-based porridge. Nutrition counseling was provided to the mothers of all children (including controls) enrolled in the trial by well-trained female 'counselors' over a total of 9 home-based counseling visits conducted monthly from 6 to 10 months of age, bimonthly at 12, 14, and 16 months of age, and a final visit at 17 months of age. A total of 11 age-specific IYCF messages were provided to the mothers.

The five groups were similar at enrollment, with small differences seen in goat/sheep ownership, exclusive breastfeeding for the first 6 months, previous 24-hour intake of some foods, and age at enrollment; 50% of households were food insecure. The prevalence of stunting at enrollment ranged from 23 to 29% in the five groups, whereas wasting prevalence was 5–6%. Adherence to supplementation was high (median 93%) in the four groups and did not differ between groups. LAZ declined with age in all five groups, and deceleration in LAZ was significantly lower (by 0.02–0.04/month) in the rice/lentil, Plumpy'doz, and chickpea groups compared to the control group at 18 months of age (table 3). WLZ decline was lower only in Plumpy'doz and chickpea groups. WSB++ was not different from the control. In children who received chickpea RUCF or Plumpy'doz, the prevalence of stunting was lower by 5–6% at 18 months (table 4). The rice/lentil, chickpea and Plumpy'doz groups had significantly greater increases in length (0.06–0.09 cm/month) and in weight (0.02–0.04 kg/month)

Table 3. Effect of complementary foods on rate of change in linear and ponderal growth among children followed from 6 to 18 months of age

	Control	Plumpy'doz	Rice/lentil	Chickpea	WSB++
Mean LAZ/month[a] (SE)	−0.06 (0.01)	−0.04 (0.01)	−0.02 (0.01)	−0.03 (0.01)	−0.05 (0.01)
Treatment effect[b] β	–	0.02	0.04	0.03	0.01
95% CI		0.004, 0.04	0.02, 0.06	0.01, 0.06	−0.02, 0.03
p value		0.02	<0.01	<0.01	0.49
Mean WLZ/month[a] (SE)	−0.22 (0.01)	−0.18 (0.01)	−0.22 (0.01)	−0.18 (0.01)	−0.20 (0.01)
Treatment effect[b] β		0.04	−0.00	0.04	0.021
95% CI		0.01, 0.06	−0.03, 0.03	0.01, 0.07	−0.01, 0.05
p value		<0.01	0.86	<0.01	0.16
Mean WAZ/month[a] (SE)	−0.10 (0.01)	−0.07 (0.01)	−0.08 (0.01)	−0.06 (0.01)	−0.08 (0.01)
Treatment effect[b] β		0.04	0.02	0.04	0.02
95% CI		0.02, 0.05	0.005, 0.04	0.03, 0.06	0.003, 0.04
p value		<0.001	0.01	<0.001	0.02
Mean length[a] (SE), cm/month	1.57 (0.02)	1.63 (0.02)	1.66 (0.02)	1.65 (0.02)	1.58 (0.02)
Treatment effect[b] β		0.06	0.09	0.08	0.01
95% CI		0.02, 0.11	0.03, 0.15	0.02, 0.14	−0.05, 0.07
p value		0.02	<0.01	0.01	0.76
Weight[a] (SE), kg/month	0.24 (0.01)	0.28 (0.01)	0.26 (0.01)	0.28 (0.01)	0.26 (0.01)
Treatment effect[b] β		0.03	0.02	0.04	0.01
95% CI		0.02, 0.05	0.003, 0.04	0.02, 0.05	−0.002, 0.03
p value		<0.001	0.02	<0.001	0.09

[a] Mixed-effect models derived monthly growth rates estimated using average marginal effects.
[b] Treatment effect β (95% CI) and p value of treatment effect derived using contrasts of average marginal effects.

compared to the control group (all $p < 0.05$). Effect sizes in the rice/lentil, chickpea, and WSB++ groups were similar to that for Plumpy'doz based on the prespecified margin of noninferiority of ±0.2 LAZ. There were no differences in the incidence of pneumonia, diarrhea, or dysentery across the intervention groups.

Conclusion

Poor-quality complementary food is a risk factor for growth retardation. RUCFs made of locally available food ingredients and conforming to standard specifications can be used to improve child growth particularly among those living in conditions of food insecurity and under social safety net mechanisms. The use of RUCFs made of locally available food ingredients can also overcome the problems of bacterial food contamination and hence reduce the risk of environmental enteropathy, which is believed to be an important cause of stunt-

Table 4. Effect of complementary foods on the prevalence of stunting, wasting, underweight, and attained length and LAZ in children at 18 months of age after 1 year of supplementation

	Control (n = 1,265)	Plumpy'doz (n = 1,344)	Rice/lentil (n = 755)	Chickpea (n = 769)	WSB++ (n = 770)
Stunting (LAZ <–2), %	44.2	40.3	43.7	39.1	44.3
Difference[a], %	–	–5.0	–2.2	–6.2	–3.9
95% CI		–8.8, –1.2	–6.5, 2.0	–10.6, –1.8	–8.1, 0.4
p value		0.01	0.30	0.006	0.07
Wasting (WLZ <–2), %	16.4	13.8	15.6	16.1	17.6
Difference[a], %	–	–2.5	–0.5	0.0	1.5
95% CI		–5.2, 0.0	–3.6, 2.6	–3.5, 3.4	–2.0, 4.9
p value		0.06	0.74	0.97	0.40
Underweight (WAZ <–2), %	39.1	32.6	38.6	34.6	40.1
Difference[a], %	–	–6.2	0.0	–5.1	–1.2
95% CI		–9.4, 3.0	–3.8, 3.8	–8.7, –1.6	–5.0, 2.5
p value		<0.001	0.99	0.005	0.52
Mean length (SD), cm	76.3 (3.0)	76.6 (2.9)	76.4 (3.0)	76.6 (3.0)	76.39 (3.0)
Difference[a], %		0.30	0.27	0.27	0.27
95% CI		0.14, 0.47	0.07, 0.47	0.05, 0.48	0.08, 0.46
p value		<0.001	<0.01	0.01	<0.01
Mean LAZ (SD)	–1.91 (1.02)	–1.80 (0.99)	–1.86 (1.01)	–1.80 (1.05)	–1.87 (1.00)
Difference[a], %*		0.10	0.07	0.08	0.10
95% CI		0.04, 0.16	0.00, 0.14	0.01, 0.16	0.03, 0.17
p value		<0.001	0.04	0.03	<0.01

[a] Using GEE linear regression analysis adjusting for baseline status.

ing [14]. Moreover, the millions of children who are underweight or are suffering from moderate acute malnutrition can also benefit if this intervention is scaled up. Certainly, the food has to be produced in bulk by the local industry. Distribution will depend upon the local context. Typically, children aged less than 5 years from food-insecure households can be targeted for complementary food supplementation. In another context, stunted or wasted children can be targeted for supplementation. In either case, nutrition counseling should be provided to underscore the importance of breastfeeding and complementary foods prepared at home under hygienic conditions.

Disclosure Statement

None of the authors received any support, financial or otherwise, from Nestec Ltd., Nestle Foundation or Nestle, for preparing this paper.

References

1 World Health Organization: Integrated Infant and Young Child Feeding Counseling: A Training Course. Participant's Manual. Geneva, WHO, 2012.

2 National Institute of Population Research and Training (NIPORT), Mitra and Associates, and ICF International. 2015. Bangladesh Demographic and Health Survey 2014: Key Indicators. Dhaka, Bangladesh, and Rockville, Maryland, USA: NIPORT, Mitra and Associates, and ICF International.

3 Khanal V, Sauer K, Zhao Y: Determinants of complementary feeding practices among Nepalese children aged 6–23 months: findings from Demographic and Health Survey 2011. BMC Pediatr 2013;13:131.

4 D'Agostino, Alexis, Anthony Begumisa, Robert Wamala, Fred Werikhe, Amanda Pomeroy, and Denis Businge. 2014. Survey Report Results on Nutrition Indicators from Six Districts in Southwest and East Central Uganda. Arlington, VA: USAID/Strengthening Partnerships, Results, and Innovations in Nutrition Globally (SPRING) Project.

5 7th five year plan FY2016-FY2020: accelerating growth, empowering citizens. General Economics Division, Planning Commission, Government of the People's Republic of Bangladesh, 2015.

6 http://aprnet.org/wp-content/uploads/2014/08/Nutrition-and-Food-Sov-in-Bangladesh.pdf (accessed on January 19, 2017).

7 Arsenault JE, Yakes EA, Hossain MB, et al: Very low adequacy of micronutrient intakes by young children and women in rural Bangladesh is primarily explained by low food intake and limited diversity. J Nutr 2013;143:197–203.

8 Yakes EA, Arsenault JE, Islam MM, et al: Intakes and breast-milk concentrations of essential fatty acids are low among Bangladeshi women with 24–48-month-old children. Br J Nutr 2011;105:1660–1670.

9 http://www.who.int/nutrition/global-target-2025/en/ (accessed on January 19, 2017).

10 WHO. Technical note: supplementary foods for the management of moderate acute malnutrition in infants and children 6–59 months of age. Geneva, World Health Organization, 2012.

11 Islam MA, Ahmed T, Faruque AS, Rahman S, Das SK, Ahmed D, Fattori V, Clarke R, Endtz HP, Cravioto A: Microbiological quality of complementary foods and its association with diarrhoeal morbidity and nutritional status of Bangladeshi children. Eur J Clin Nutr 2012; 66:1242–1246.

12 Ahmed T, Choudhury N, Hossain I, et al: Development and acceptability testing of ready-to-use supplementary food made from locally available food ingredients in Bangladesh. BMC Pediatr 2014;14:164.

13 Christian P, Shaikh S, Shamim AA, et al: Effect of fortified complementary food supplementation on child growth in rural Bangladesh: a cluster-randomized trial. Int J Epidemiol 2015;44:1862–1876.

14 Petri WA Jr, Naylor C, Haque R. Environmental enteropathy and malnutrition: do we know enough to intervene? BMC Med 2014; 12:187.

Black RE, Makrides M, Ong KK (eds): Complementary Feeding: Building the Foundations for a Healthy Life. Nestlé Nutr Inst Workshop Ser, vol 87, pp 115–129, (DOI: 10.1159/000449210)
Nestec Ltd., Vevey/S. Karger AG., Basel, © 2017

Fortification of Complementary Foods: A Review of Products and Program Delivery

Lynnette M. Neufeld[a] · Saskia J.M. Osendarp[b] · Wendy Gonzalez[a]

[a]Global Alliance for Improved Nutrition, Geneva, Switzerland; [b]Independent Consultant OsendarpNutrition, Berkel & Rodenrijs, The Netherlands

Abstract

Fortified complementary foods (FCF) and home fortificants – single-sachet micronutrient powders (MNP) or small-quantity lipid-based nutrient supplements (SQ-LNS) to be added to a child's food immediately before consumption – have been shown to be efficacious to improve the micronutrient status and some functional outcomes in children 6–23 months of age. The objective of this chapter is to describe and discuss the latest advances related to the composition and delivery of FCF products, including home and commercial fortification. For FCF and MNPs, there is guidance to ensure that products are safe and aligned with recommendations. Impact, however, can be achieved only if adequate attention is paid to program design and implementation, including the choice of the delivery platform, and ensuring availability, accessibility, acceptability, coverage, and utilization by the target population. Well-targeted programs such as social protection programs, health services, community-based vendors (referred to as market based), child health weeks, and emergency programs have all been used as delivery platforms for FCF and MNPs. To date, guidance for formulation and programmatic experience with the distribution of SQ-LNS is limited. An in-depth understanding of the local context and culture, and the design and implementation of program components, including behavior change interventions that respond to those, can increase program coverage and product utilization. Using rigorous process evaluation would permit to adapt programs to increase their potential for impact, strengthen the evidence related to how programs work, and allow the development of program guidance to increase effective implementation.

Introduction

The need for nutrient-dense complementary foods in addition to continued breastfeeding as of the 6th month of life has long been recognized. The functional consequences of inadequate breast and complementary feeding include impaired growth and cognitive and motor development – topics that have been addressed by a number of papers in this series. Even where energy requirements for adequate growth and development are met, a number of essential nutrients may be inadequate in commonly consumed complementary foods [1], and micronutrient deficiency is often high in children 6–24 months of age [2].

Unless foods of animal source are regularly included in the diet, it is difficult for infants and young children to consume sufficient quantities of iron and zinc from unfortified complementary foods [3]. Where resources constrain access to diverse diets, other nutrients may also be limited in common complementary foods [3]. Linear programming methods, particularly the Optifood and Cost of the Diet tools, have permitted an optimization of the use of local ingredients to improve the quality of complementary foods in the home. Some studies have also shown the potential of germination and fermentation to increase the density and bioavailability of certain nutrients in complementary foods. Requirements for a number of nutrients can be consistently met through optimizing the use of available local ingredients, (e.g., proteins, vitamin A, vitamin C), whereas those of others are rarely adequate (e.g., iron and zinc) (table 1). Ensuring adequate nutrient density of complementary foods may be prohibitive for reasons of availability and/or affordability in many contexts [3, 4].

Where needed, nutrient intake of infants and young children can be increased using nutrient supplements, but adherence to such products is often low [5], and some have raised concerns of safety [6]. There is some evidence that fortification of oil can improve intake [7] and vitamin A status [8] as can the consumption of iodine from iodized salt [9]. The contribution of other nutrients from fortified staple foods, such as iron or zinc from flour or rice, is likely to be minimal due to the limited gastric capacity of infants and young children.

The nutrient density of complementary foods can be increased through fortification, either commercially at the time of production or through the addition of nutrients in the home before consuming (referred to as home fortification). The objective of this paper is to describe and discuss the latest advances related to the composition and delivery of fortified complementary food (FCF) products, including home and commercial fortification. We will begin with a brief description of the products, including the latest guidelines and specifications for their development and production. We will then review the delivery of home fortificants [micronutrient powders (MNP) and small-quantity lipid-based nu-

Table 1. Nutrient content of complementary foods can be substantially improved by optimizing use of local foods, but some gaps remain

Consistently feasible to reach adequacy	Inadequate in some scenarios	Usually inadequate
Protein	Thiamine	Iron
Vitamin B_{12}	Riboflavin	Zinc
Vitamin C	Folate	
Vitamin A	Calcium	

trient supplements (SQ-LNS)] and FCFs through multiple program models, focusing on the many aspects needed for programs to be successful. The latter is organized across the pathway by which such programs can have impact on functional outcomes, including availability, accessibility, acceptability, coverage, and utilization, drawing on experience from programs and research in low- and middle-income countries.

Home Fortification

Home fortification refers to the addition of nutrients to foods immediately before consumption. The term was coined soon after the invention of MNPs or single-serving sachets originally containing 3 micronutrients. MNPs were developed as an alternative to iron syrup for the treatment and later prevention of anemia [5]. They are equally efficacious to address iron deficiency and anemia, with some evidence suggesting that they may be more acceptable [10]. Later products included up to 15 micronutrients, and their potential as a way to improve the quality of complementary foods has been recognized [11]. There is little evidence, however, for outcomes beyond anemia and iron deficiency, and World Health Organization (WHO) recommendations at this time focus on anemia reduction [12].

Building on the success of ready-to-use therapeutic foods for the treatment of acute malnutrition, SQ-LNS was designed to provide a small daily dose of essential nutrients in a lipid-based paste. Similar to MNPs, the product is added to single servings of complementary foods immediately before consumption. In addition to micronutrients, SQ-LNS provides energy, protein (usually milk), essential fatty acids, and calcium. A number of efficacy trials have now demonstrated the potential of SQ-LNS to improve the energy and nutrient density of complementary foods as well as some functional outcomes, although the impact on growth and development is mixed and seems to be context specific [13–15].

Table 2. Recommended composition of MNPs for children 6–59 months of age[a]

Micronutrient	Amount in MNP
Vitamin A (RE), µg	400
Vitamin D_3, µg	5.0
Vitamin E (TE), mg	5.0
Vitamin C, mg	30
Thiamine (vitamin B_1), mg	0.5
Riboflavin (vitamin B_2), mg	0.5
Niacin, mg	6.0
Vitamin B_6, mg	0.5
Vitamin B_{12}, µg	0.9
Folic acid, µg	90
Iron, mg	10
Zinc, mg	4.1
Copper, mg	0.56
Selenium, µg	17
Iodine, µg	90

[a] Reproduced from HF-TAG MNP Composition Manual [16].

To date, SQ-LNS has been a sweet product, and a number of trials have reported the preference of children (and caregivers) for direct consumption rather than addition to regular complementary foods [15].

Resources exist that identify good practice for the development and composition of MNPs. The Home Fortification Technical Advisory Group (HF-TAG), an ad hoc group of experts who provide technical support to countries and organizations on design, implementation, and evaluation of home fortification programs, has published a composition manual and a manufacturing manual [16, 17]. Table 2 shows the content of standard MNP sachets recommended by the HF-TAG [16]. At this time, no similar guidance manuals have been developed for SQ-LNS.

The revised Codex [Guidelines on formulated complementary foods for older infants and young children (CAC/GL 8-1991)], adopted in July 2013, now includes SQ-LNS as a separate food category but does not refer to MNPs. Both MNPs and SQ-LNS were also excluded from the recent draft guidance on ending inappropriate promotion of foods for infants and young children (WHO EB 138/8, January 15, 2016) as they are not considered 'foods'. Whether they are registered as food, food supplement, or medicine is dependent on the laws in each country and has varied. The WHO recommends that many of the principles in the guidance related to the promotion of foods, including those concerning adherence to national and global standards for nutrient levels, safety and quality, should be applied to such products. Messages indicating their use for infants less than 6 months of age are appropriately prohibited.

Fortified Complementary Foods[1]

The nutrient content that should be delivered by complementary foods varies widely, depending on the concentration of each nutrient in breast milk and other commonly consumed foods. The micronutrients for which most of the requirements should come from complementary foods are iron, zinc, and vitamin B_6 [18] due to their low content in breast milk.

The Subgroup on Formulations of the Ten Year Strategy to Reduce Vitamin and Mineral Deficiencies, Maternal, Infant, and Young Child Nutrition Working Group reviewed the literature on recommendations for FCFs [19]. FCFs that have been successful in improving dietary intakes and some health outcomes (micronutrient status and/or growth) have generally included cereals or maltodextrin, a nutrient-dense fat source such as full-fat soy flour or whole-milk powder, high-quality protein (if limited in the diet, estimated at 5–15% calories as protein), whole or reduced-fat milk, and micronutrients.

Complementary foods should be semisolid or solid in order to assist transition from a liquid diet to a regular diet and should not be fed from a bottle, which might interfere with breastfeeding. Products should ideally be precooked or instant in order to improve ease of preparation, both in time and fuel needed. Manufacturing processes that assist in lowering the levels of antinutrient factors are desirable as these can inhibit the bioavailability of nutrients (e.g., phytate and tannins) or interfere with digestion (e.g., α-amylase inhibitors and protease inhibitors such as trypsin and saponins) [19]. The marketing of all complementary feeding products should comply with the International Code of Marketing of Breast Milk Substitutes and subsequent Resolutions by the World Health Assembly.

The energy density of FCFs should be at least 0.8 kcal/g of product served [20], and a higher energy density is preferable. A minimum protein-energy ratio of 6% in complementary foods has been recommended by Lutter and Dewey [20], but in order to fulfil the essential amino acid needs, the absolute amount required will depend on the protein source and energy content of the product.

[1] For the purposes of this paper, we refer to fortified food products designed for children as of 6 months of age (and usually until 23 months of age) as FCFs. Other terms commonly used are fortified blended foods, complementary food supplements, and fortified infant porridge, among others.

Inclusion of small amounts of milk products in FCF has been suggested to be beneficial for growth. The biological basis for this effect is not known and may be related to the presence of calcium, phosphorus, and magnesium, or specific amino acids such as lysine, which are abundant in dairy foods and may have growth-promoting abilities. In addition, the intake of cow's milk may also stimulate insulin-like growth factor 1 secretion, which has a direct effect on linear growth [21].

Breast milk is an abundant source of lipids, and the energy content from fat in breast milk ranges from 45 to 55% of energy [22]. From 6 months to 3 years of age, fat intake should be reduced gradually from 40–60 to 30–35% of total energy, with the higher end of the range referable for more physically active children [23]. To facilitate that transition, a range of 30–45% of the total energy intake from dietary fat per day from complementary foods has been recommended for children from 6 to 23 months of age [1, 22]. Requirements for the essential fatty acids include that at least 3–4.5% of total energy should come from linoleic acid (ω-6 fatty acids) and ≥0.5% of total energy from α-linolenic acid (ω-3 fatty acids) [24].

The WHO/FAO (Food and Agriculture Organization of the United States) have established levels of reference nutrient intake [25] and upper intake levels for micronutrients, which are based on the requirements for healthy children. Recommended fortification levels for complementary foods are summarized in table 3 [20]. When a product is targeted to the entire age range, the higher level of the recommended nutrient intake is typically recommended, as this will meet the needs of all groups as long as it remains below the upper intake levels for all age groups.

There are concerns on providing excess iron to iron-replete children, particularly those living in poor hygienic and sanitation conditions, because the daily provision of supplemental doses of iron may alter the composition of the gut microflora and exacerbate the presence and severity of infections, including malaria and diarrhea [26]. Because of these concerns, recent recommendations for FCFs suggest limiting the iron content of one serving to 50% of the reference nutrient intake. Recommended iron compounds include ferrous sulfate, encapsulated ferrous sulfate, ferrous fumarate, and electrolytic iron [27], or ferrous sulfate, ferrous fumarate, and ferric pyrophosphate [28]. Sodium iron EDTA (NaFeEDTA) may have advantages for bioavailability, but its use may be limited due to the need to keep EDTA intake below the upper intake level [29].

Delivery Models

In high-income populations, the use of FCFs is almost universal [30], and a variety of products are available on the market at diverse prices and designed to meet specific needs or desires (e.g., kosher or organic). Programs targeted

Table 3. Desired micronutrient density of consumed complementary foods (per 100 kcal) per age group, assuming an average intake and composition of breast milk[a, b]

Nutrient	Age group		
	6–8 months	9–11 months	12–23 months
Vitamin A, μg RE	31	30	23
Vitamin D, μg	2.5	1.5	0.9
Vitamin E, mg	–	–	–
Vitamin K, μg	3.3	2	1.2
Vitamin B_1/thiamine, mg	0.08	0.06	0.07
Vitamin B_2/riboflavin, mg	0.08	0.06	0.06
Vitamin B_3/niacin, mg	1.5	1	0.9
Vitamin B_5/pantothenic acid, mg	0.2	0.1	0.1
Vitamin B_6/pyridoxine, mg	0.12	0.08	0.08
Vitamin B_9/folic acid, μg	11	9	21
Vitamin B_{12}/cobalamin, μg	0.07	0.08	0.12
Vitamin C, mg	1.5	1.7	1.5
Calcium, mg	105	74	63
Iodine, μg	45	30	16.4
Iron, mg[a]	4.5	3	1
Zinc, mg[a]	1.6	1.1	0.6
Copper, mg	0.04	0.02	0.04
Selenium, μg	0	0	0.5
Choline, mg	81	53	76
Magnesium, mg	19	13	9
Manganese, μg	4	3	2
Phosphorus, mg	114	70	26
Potassium, mg	129	84	69
Sodium, mg	74	53	54

[a] Based on medium bioavailability.

[b] Reproduced with permission from Lutter and Dewey [20].

at low-income populations in high-income countries may include coupons for the purchase of FCFs, such as the Women, Infants and Children program in the United States (https://www.health.ny.gov/publications/4008/#wic11).

In low- and middle-income countries, such products are often available in urban settings but may be less accessible to the poor or those living in rural or isolated areas. The willingness of businesses to develop and distribute more affordable FCFs or SQ-LNS may be limited unless risks related to demand creation and low margins can be mitigated [31, 32]. Some programs have attempted to overcome these barriers by creating public-private partnerships, bringing together business, nongovernmental organizations, and academia to

Table 4. Qualitative assessment of the four platforms according to the seven performance criteria based on the cumulative evidence[a]

Criteria	Agriculture	Health	Market based	Social protection
Targeting	Good	Good	Good	Good
Interventions	Good	Good	Good	Good
Implementation	Needs improvement	Needs improvement	Needs improvement	Needs improvement
Utilization	Needs improvement	Needs improvement	Need more information	Needs improvement
Impact	Need more information	Good	Need more information	Good
Coverage	Needs improvement	Needs improvement	Need more information	Good
Sustainability	Need more information	Need more information	Need more information	Good

[a] Reproduced with permission from Olney et al. [36].

ensure that the composition and production of the products meet current standards but still remain affordable for the intended target population and generate demand simultaneous with improving availability and quality [31, 33].

Many programs aim to improve the nutrition and health outcomes of children through the free or subsidized distribution of FCFs and/or MNPs. Over 60 countries globally have implemented MNP programs [34]. Small-scale programs that distribute SQ-LNS have been implemented in Guatemala and Burundi (evaluation results forthcoming). In Latin America, FCFs have been widely commercially available and used for many years, and in a number of countries in the region, they are distributed free of cost to low-income households [35].

The choice of a potential delivery platform for such programs depends on the population to be reached and the alternatives already available to reach them, among other factors. The potential and experience of diverse platforms, including agriculture, social protection programs, health services, and community-based vendors (referred to as market based), have been described previously (table 4) [36]. The authors stress the importance of delivering efficacious interventions via these platforms and highlight a number of examples including FCFs and MNPs. Targeting, defined as reaching pregnant women and children 6–23 months of age, is an important strength of these platforms.

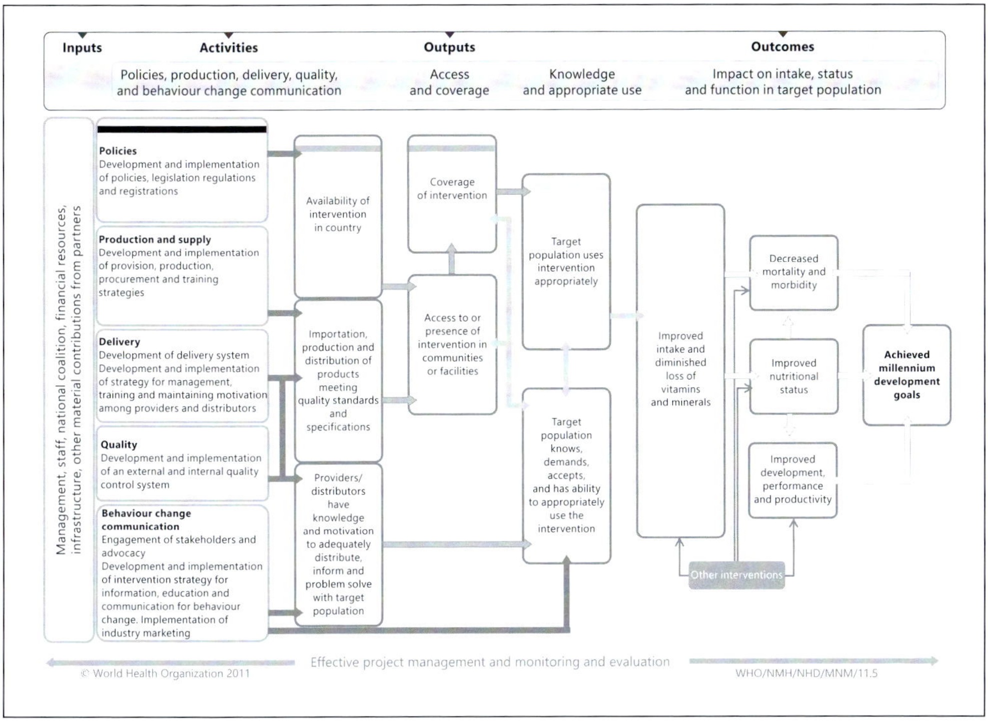

Fig. 1. WHO/CDC logic model for micronutrient interventions in public health (reproduced with permission from De-Regil et al. [37]).

Whatever the delivery platform, the ultimate success of a program will depend on the consistent supply and high coverage and utilization by those with potential to benefit. Although intuitive, the many considerations necessary to achieve this have often been inadequately taken into consideration in program design and implementation. The next section will review related evidence and program experience.

Components of Successful Programs

The ultimate goal of home and commercial fortification is to improve the health, growth, and development of young children, mediated through improved intake and utilization of nutrients, but many factors must be in place for programs to be impactful. To facilitate a common understanding of the processes and actions required for successful programs, the WHO and the Centers for Disease Control and Prevention (CDC) developed the WHO/CDC logic model for micronutrient interventions in public health (fig. 1) [37]. Biological impact of any FCF will be dependent on the extent to which that product meets nutritional needs and is consumed regularly by those with a potential to benefit (i.e., that it is appropriately targeted). This model shows that in addition to the selection of the delivery platform, well-functioning logistics and enabling environment with appropriate policies are also required to ensure product quality, availability, accessibility, and coverage. Effective behavior change interventions (BCI) can facilitate acceptance and promote adequate adherence and appropriate use [37] while promoting appropriate infant feeding more broadly, including breastfeeding.

Similar to the fortification of staple foods [38], the setting and enforcement of composition and quality standards for FCFs and home fortificants are a critical part of program planning. For standardized products such as MNPs, the existence of concrete guidance and procurement from global suppliers (i.e., UNICEF Supply Division) has facilitated quality assurance.

A number of models have been used for FCF production, from small-scale production by community organizations to large-scale commercial production. In some countries, technical support with or without additional incentives has been used with some success to strengthen local small- and medium-scale industry capacity to produce high-quality FCF at low cost [31, 33]. In Latin America, with large-scale distribution through social programs, products have been produced by medium- to large-scale industry for many decades. This has a number of advantages, including potentially better acceptance due to the prestige of known producers, competition for government procurement contracts, and possibly sustainability if products are also sold on the market [35].

Delivery through well-targeted existing programs can greatly increase access and coverage [36]. In Mexico, for example, the inclusion of a FCF through the conditional cash transfer program resulted in high coverage to the segment of the population with the highest prevalence of stunting and a measurable improvement in nutrient intake [39]. MNPs have been delivered through multiple program models that are well targeted to reach low-income and rural populations, including community-based health workers and health facilities in Nepal [40], community sales agents in Kenya [41] and Bangladesh [42], and child health weeks in Nigeria [43], among others.

Even in very well-targeted programs, impact will be dependent on the extent to which products (and associated services) are accepted and used by the population. Both supply and demand side challenges were reported in most of the MNP programs mentioned above. Fostering acceptance and stimulating demand for complementary feeding products are most effective when cultural and other barriers, and facilitators to acceptance and appropriate use, are well

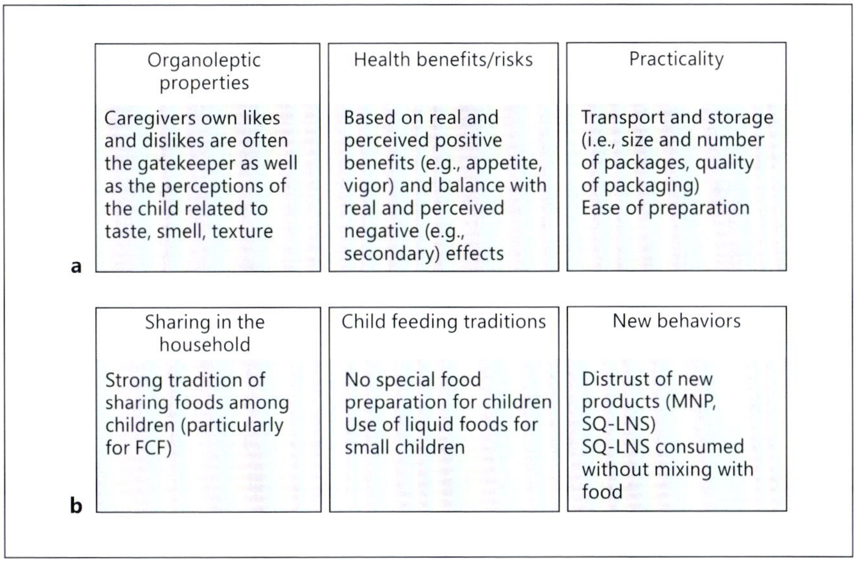

Fig. 2. Common barriers and factors that facilitate acceptance (**a**) and utilization (**b**) of MNPs and FCFs.

understood and used to guide the development of BCI [44]. From the example mentioned in Mexico, the strong cultural tradition of sharing foods among all children in the home proved difficult to modify resulting in modifications to the program to adapt to this. Although specific supply and demand barriers and enhancers are context specific, there are a number of common themes that emerge in reviewing studies in multiple contexts. For example, organoleptic properties, perceived health benefits and risks, and practicality are consistently important to influence acceptance (fig. 2a). Utilization is highly and consistently influenced by overall child feeding practices and sharing of the product with other household members, as well as the extent to which new and or complex behaviors are required to adopt the product (fig. 2b).

BCI for home fortification programs may require additional considerations to support sustained adherence and appropriate use of the product [45]. For instance, unlike FCF, which are often an adaptation of existing foods for children, MNPs and SQ-LNS are new products. The nutrition problems they seek to address (e.g., inadequate micronutrient intake) may not be perceived or prioritized by the caregiver, and the products themselves may be received with caution. Inadequate attention to the identification of such issues in formative research and strategies to address them, for example, resulted in very low utilization of MNPs in one project implemented in a refugee camp [46]. When products are provided to the household, an in-depth understanding of the pattern of utilization, including both under- and overutilization and sharing, is needed to identify potential benefits and risks of programs [47].

For all programs, effective monitoring that has been purposefully designed to provide continual feedback for program improvement is essential, and a detailed manual to support this has been developed [48]. The manual, although developed for MNPs, is applicable for all programs that include complementary feeding products. Process evaluation to assess and improve program performance is also critical, but there are still few examples of comprehensive process evaluations in the published literature. In Nigeria, a number of challenges were identified, including issues of supply chain, training, and sufficient time allocation for BCI [43]. Implementation research, for example in Nepal comparing the rollout and coverage achieved as a result of different delivery models [40], identified challenges to achieving coverage suggesting a need for different delivery channels.

Summary and Conclusions

FCFs and home fortification provide a programmatically viable alternative to improve the quality of diets for children 6–23 months of age. A number of programs have sought to increase their availability and/or affordability by working directly with industry (from small to large scale), but challenges remain to create viable business models for the production of complementary feeding products.

Many public programs target populations at high risk of inadequate dietary nutrient intake in infants with free or subsidized distribution of complementary feeding products. The free distribution of FCFs is common across the Latin-American region, and many countries around the world are now distributing MNPs. At this time, the use of SQ-LNS in programs is still very limited.

There is ample guidance to ensure the production of commodities/products meet safety standards and nutrient requirements, as well as guidance on program monitoring and implementation. The selection and development of the product itself is critical, but the impact on nutritional status and functional outcomes will be achieved only if adequate attention is paid to program implementation. In this chapter, we use the WHO/CDC generic logic model for programs to guide a review of critical program components, particularly the choice of the delivery platform and factors that influence product supply, demand, and utilization by the target population. For FCFs, there are a number of challenges that must be overcome, including lack of perception of need for the products and sharing of products in the home. These and other challenges can only be overcome with program components, including BCI, grounded and developed with an in-depth understanding of the local context and culture. This highlights the need for formative research to be used to guide the design of all programs.

Process evaluation and implementation research are tools that should also be used in all programs to track performance – i.e., the quality of implementation in comparison to design, and provide specific recommendations to improve the quality of design and implementation. Using rigorous designs and ensuring high-quality research would strengthen the evidence related to how programs work and permit the development of program guidance to increase effective implementation.

Disclosure Statement

The authors declare that no financial or other conflict of interest exists in relation to the contents of the chapter.

References

1 Dewey KG, Brown KH: Update on technical issues concerning complementary feeding of young children in developing countries and implications for intervention programs. Food Nutr Bull 2003;24:5–28.

2 Black RE: Global Distribution and Disease Burden Related to Micronutrient Deficiencies. Nestlé Nutr Inst Workshop Ser. Basel, Karger, 2014, vol 78, pp 21–28.

3 Osendarp SJM, Broersen B, van Liere MJ, et al: Complementary feeding diets made of local foods can be optimized, but additional interventions will be needed to meet iron and zinc requirements in 6- to 23-month-old children in low- and middle-income countries. Food Nutr Bull 2016;pii: 0379572116655239.

4 Baldi G, Martini E, Catharina M, et al: Cost of the Diet (CoD) tool: first results from Indonesia and applications for policy discussion on food and nutrition security. Food Nutr Bull 2013;34(2 suppl):S35–S42.

5 Zlotkin S, Antwi KY, Schauer C, Yeung G: Use of microencapsulated iron(II) fumarate sprinkles to prevent recurrence of anaemia in infants and young children at high risk. Bull World Health Organ 2003;81:108–115.

6 Raiten DJ, Neufeld LM, De-Regil L-M, et al: Integration to implementation and the micronutrient forum: a coordinated approach for global nutrition. Case study application: safety and effectiveness of iron interventions. Adv Nutr 2016;7:135–148.

7 Friesen VM: Assessing coverage of large-scale food fortification interventions: Fortification Assessment Coverage Toolkit (FACT) results and implications. Micronutrient Forum 2016, Cancun, October 24–28, 2016.

8 Sandjaja, Jus'at I, Jahari AB, et al: Vitamin A-fortified cooking oil reduces vitamin A deficiency in infants, young children and women: results from a programme evaluation in Indonesia. Public Health Nutr 2015;18: 2511–2522.

9 Aburto NJ, Abudou M, Candeias V, Wu T: Effect and Safety of Salt Iodization to Prevent Iodine Deficiency Disorders: A Systematic Review with Meta-Analyses. Geneva, WHO, 2014.

10 De-Regil LM, Suchdev PS, Vist GE, et al: Home fortification of foods with multiple micronutrient powders for health and nutrition in children under two years of age. Cochrane Database Syst Rev 2011;9:CD008959.

11 de Pee S, Irizarry L, Kraemer K, Jefferds MED: Micronutrient powder interventions: the basis for current programming guidance and needs for additional knowledge and experience; in de Pee S, Flores-Ayala R, Van Hees J, et al (eds): Home Fortification with Micronutrition Powders (MNP). Basel, Sight and Life, 2013, pp 51–56.
12 World Health Organization. Guideline: Use of Multiple Micronutrient Powders for Home Fortification of Foods Consumed by Infants and Children 6–23 Months of Age. Geneva, WHO, 2011.
13 Hess SY, Abbeddou S, Jimenez EY, et al: Small-quantity lipid-based nutrient supplements, regardless of their zinc content, increase growth and reduce the prevalence of stunting and wasting in young Burkinabe children: a cluster-randomized trial. PLoS One 2015;10:e0122242.
14 Maleta KM, Phuka J, Alho L, et al: Provision of 10–40 g/d lipid-based nutrient supplements from 6 to 18 months of age does not prevent linear growth faltering in Malawi. J Nutr 2015;145:1909–1915.
15 Arimond M, Zeilani M, Jungjohann S, et al: Considerations in developing lipid-based nutrient supplements for prevention of undernutrition: experience from the International Lipid-Based Nutrient Supplements (iLiNS) Project. Matern Child Nutr 2015;11:31–61.
16 Home Fortification Technical Advisory Group: Manual on Micronutrient Powder (MNPs) Composition. Geneva, Home Fortification Technical Advisory Group, 2013.
17 Home Fortification Technical Advisory Group: UNIDO. Quality Manual on Micronutrient Powders – A Guiding Document. Geneva/Vienna, Home Fortification Technical Advisory Group/United Nations Industrial Development Organization, 2014.
18 Dewey K: Complementary feeding; in Caballero B, Allen L, Prentice A (eds): Encyclopedia of Human Nutrition. Amsterdam, Elsevier, 2005, pp 465–470.
19 Young Child Nutrition Working Group: Formulation Subgroup: Formulations for fortified complementary foods and supplements: review of successful products for improving the nutritional status of infants and young children. Food Nutr Bull 2009;30(2 suppl): S239–S255.
20 Lutter CK, Dewey KG: Proposed nutrient composition for fortified complementary foods. J Nutr 2003;133:3011S–3020S.
21 Fleischer Michaelsen K, Hoppe C, Lauritzen L, Mølgaard C: Whole Cow's Milk: Why, What and When?; in Agostoni C, Brunser O (eds): Issues in Complementary. Feeding Nestlé Nutr Work Ser Paediatr Program. Philadelphia, Lippincott Williams & Wilkins, 2007, vol 60, pp 201–216; discussion 216–219.
22 World Health Organization: Complementary Feeding of Young Children in Developing Countries: A Review of Current Scientific Knowledge. Geneva, WHO, 1998.
23 Uauy R, Castillo C: Lipid requirements of infants: implications for nutrient composition of fortified complementary foods. J Nutr 2003;133:2962S–2972S.
24 Fats and fatty acids in human nutrition. Proceedings of the Joint FAO/WHO Expert Consultation. November 10-14, 2008. Geneva, Switzerland. Ann Nutr Metab 2009;55: 5–300.
25 WHO/FAO: Vitamin and Mineral Requirements in Human Nutrition, ed 2. Geneva, WHO, 2004.
26 Jaeggi T, Kortman GAM, Moretti D, et al: Iron fortification adversely affects the gut microbiome, increases pathogen abundance and induces intestinal inflammation in Kenyan infants. Gut 2015;64:731–742.
27 World Health Organization, Food and Agricultural Organization of the United Nations: Guidelines on Food Fortification with Micronutrients. Geneva, WHO, 2006.
28 Davidsson L, Sarker SA, Jamil KA, et al: Regular consumption of a complementary food fortified with ascorbic acid and ferrous fumarate or ferric pyrophosphate is as useful as ferrous sulfate in maintaining hemoglobin concentrations >105 g/l in young Bangladeshi children. Am J Clin Nutr 2009;89:1815–2180.
29 Yang Z, Siekmann J, Schofield D: Fortifying complementary foods with NaFeEDTA – considerations for developing countries. Matern Child Nutr 2011;7(suppl 3):123–128.
30 Grummer-Strawn LM, Scanlon KS, Fein SB: Infant feeding and feeding transitions during the first year of life. Pediatrics 2008; 122(suppl):S36–S42.

31 van Liere MJ, Frega R, Tariton D, Schofield D: Infant and Young Child Nutrition: Paper 1. Improving Complementary Feeding: Assessing Public and Private Sector Business Models. Geneva, Global Alliance for Improved Nutrition, 2015.
32 Segrè J, Winnard K, Abrha TH, et al: Willingness to pay for lipid-based nutrient supplements for young children in four urban sites of Ethiopia. Matern Child Nutr 2015;11:16–30.
33 Bruyeron O, Denizeau M, Berger J, Trèche S: Marketing complementary foods and supplements in Burkina Faso, Madagascar, and Vietnam: lessons learned from the Nutridev program. Food Nutr Bull 2010;31:S154–S167.
34 United Nations Children's Fund: Multiple Micronutrient Powder Supply & Outlook. Copenhagen, UNICEF, 2014.
35 Rivera JA, Lutter CK: The potential role of processed complementary food in Latin America; in Martorell R, Haschke F (eds): Nutrition and Growth. Nestlé Nutr Work Ser Paediatr Program. Philadelphia, Lippincott Williams & Wilkins, 2000, vol 47, pp 281–304.
36 Olney DK, Rawat R, Ruel MT: Identifying potential programs and platforms to deliver multiple micronutrient interventions. J Nutr 2012;142:178S–185S.
37 De-Regil LM, Peña-Rosas JP, Flores-Ayala R, et al: Development and use of the generic WHO/CDC logic model for vitamin and mineral interventions in public health programmes. Public Health Nutr 2014;17:634–639.
38 Luthringer CL, Rowe LA, Vossenaar M, Garrett GS: Regulatory monitoring of fortified foods: identifying barriers and good practices. Glob Heal Sci Pract 2015;3:446–461.
39 Ramirez-Silva I, Rivera JA, Leroy JL, Neufeld LM: The Oportunidades program's fortified food supplement, but not improvements in the home diet, increased the intake of key micronutrients in rural Mexican children aged 12–59 months. J Nutr 2013;143:656–663.
40 Jefferds MED, Mirkovic KR, Subedi GR, et al: Predictors of micronutrient powder sachet coverage in Nepal. Matern Child Nutr 2015; 11:77–89.
41 Suchdev PS, Ruth LJ, Woodruff BA, et al: Selling Sprinkles micronutrient powder reduces anemia, iron deficiency, and vitamin A deficiency in young children in Western Kenya: a cluster-randomized controlled trial. Am J Clin Nutr 2012;95:1223–1230.
42 Afsana K, Haque MR, Sobhan S, Shahin SA: BRAC's experience in scaling-up MNP in Bangladesh. Asia Pac J Clin Nutr 2014;23: 377–384.
43 Korenromp EL, Adeosun O, Adegoke F, et al: Micronutrient powder distribution through Maternal, Neonatal and Child Health Weeks in Nigeria: process evaluation of feasibility and use. Public Health Nutr 2015;19:1882–1892.
44 Pelto GH, Martin SL, Van Liere M, Fabrizio CS: The scope and practice of behaviour change communication to improve infant and young child feeding in low- and middle-income countries: results of a practitioner study in international development organizations. Matern Child Nutr 2016;12:229–244.
45 Jefferds ME, Irizarry L, Timmer A, Tripp K: UNICEF-CDC global assessment of home fortification interventions 2011: current status, new directions, and implications for policy and programmatic guidance. Food Nutr Bull 2013;34:434–443.
46 Kodish S, Rah J, Kraemer K: Understanding low usage of micronutrient powder in the Kakuma Refugee Camp, Kenya: findings from a qualitative study. Food Nutr Bull 2011;32:292–303.
47 Kodish SR, Aburto NJ, Nseluke Hambayi M, et al: Patterns and determinants of small-quantity LNS utilization in rural Malawi and Mozambique: considerations for interventions with specialized nutritious foods. Matern Child Nutr, Epub ahead of print.
48 Home Fortification Technical Advisory Group. A Manual for Developing and Implementing Monitoring Systems for Home Fortification Interventions. Geneva, Home Fortification Technical Advisory Group, 2013.

Black RE, Makrides M, Ong KK (eds): Complementary Feeding: Building the Foundations for a Healthy Life. Nestlé Nutr Inst Workshop Ser, vol 87, pp 131–138, (DOI: 10.1159/000448962)
Nestec Ltd., Vevey/S. Karger AG., Basel, © 2017

Ying Yang Bao: Improving Complementary Feeding for Chinese Infants in Poor Regions

Junsheng Huo

Institute for Nutrition and Health, Chinese Center for Disease Control and Prevention, Beijing, China

Abstract

Ying Yang Bao (YYB), a complementary food supplement, has helped to rapidly improve the nutrition status of infants and young children in poor rural regions in China. The first YYB study was performed in 2001 by the International Life Sciences Institute, the Chinese Centers for Disease Control and Prevention, and Nestlé. In 2008, the establishment of national standards for complementary food supplements stimulated implementation of about 15 nutrition intervention projects in poor rural counties in which YYB was applied to infants and young children as home fortification for complementary feeding. Data were accumulated in different studies and showed that YYB enhanced the growth of infants with respect to both anthropometry and cognition, and decreased anemia prevalence significantly in infants aged 6–24 months. The Chinese government has launched a project named Improving Children's Nutrition in Poor Rural Regions in 2012. The project has covered more than 4 million infants aged 6–24 months in 341 counties in 21 provinces in western and middle regions by the end of 2015. This nutrition intervention in early life is rather an opportunity for a better later life. The YYB program in China might present an example for developing countries aiming to improve nutrition in early life.

Introduction

Ying Yang Bao (YYB), 12 g per sachet, is a soy bean powder-based complementary food supplement containing vitamin A, D, B_1, B_2, B_6, folic acid, calcium, iron, and zinc. YYB can be used as home fortification product of complementary foods and added to porridge, noodles, and other homemade complementary foods. The aim of YYB was to prevent infants and young children (IYCN) from malnutrition, especially in rural China, where the prevalence of stunting and anemia is significantly higher than in urban regions. Inadequate supply of high-quality protein and micronutrients during the complementary feeding period has been considered as one of the main reasons for stunting and anemia [1, 2]. The YYB project has rapidly developed in poor rural counties as a government action aiming to eliminate malnutrition. This paper reviews the development of YYB and the data accumulated regarding its nutritional effect.

Development of Ying Yang Bao

During the 1990s, more than 100 million children under 5 years of age were undernourished in China. Most of these children lived in poor rural areas. This inacceptable situation has attracted the attention of Madam Chen Chunming, the founder of the Chinese Academy of Preventive Medicine. Together with her team, she is continuously striving to improve nutrition and promote food fortification for undernourished infants and young children. Madam Chen Chunming has initiated research to study the effects of home fortification; during this intervention (from 2001 to 2003), sachets of complementary food which contained soy bean powder enriched with micronutrients were provided to infants (1 sachet per day per infant). The results showed that the nutrition status and cognitive scores were improved in the test group, and the differences compared with other groups (rice powder group and control group) were significant. The cost-benefit analysis of the study suggested that the home fortification with enriched soy bean powder was highly acceptable in terms of social feasibility as an approach to improve public nutrition. Lately, the nutrient-enriched soy bean powder was habitually called Ying Yang Bao (YYB), a Chinese translation meaning nutrient sachets. Nestlé developed the YYB product and donated the product for the intervention in Madam Chen's study [3].

In 2007, the Institute of Nutrition and Food Safety (INFS) of the Chinese Centers for Disease Control and Prevention (CDC) advised the Ministry of Health (MOH) to supply YYB in poor rural areas as a public nutrition promotion project, and the proposal was verified by the MOH in 2008. Supported by the MOH and the Global Alliance for Improved Nutrition (GAIN), the INFS started YYB promotion projects in Huguan County, Changzhi County, and Meixian County in Shanxi Province and Shaanxi Province. Nutritional information on YYB was distributed through Mother and Child Health Care Centers via doctor consultants combined with brochures and posts. Local consumers could buy YYB products from stores which were specifically involved in this governmental project. Meanwhile, the Food Fortification Office

Table 1. Nutrition formula of YYB used in the project to improve child nutrition in poor regions

	(12 g/sachet)
Protein, g	3
Iron, mg	7.5
Zinc, mg	5
Calcium, mg	200
Vitamin A, μg	250
Vitamin D, μg	5
Vitamin B_1, mg	0.5
Vitamin B_2, mg	0.5
Vitamin B_{12}, μg	0.5
Folic acid, μg	75

Other ingredients were soy bean powder.

(FFO) of the Chinese CDC started to establish national standards for YYB supported by ILSI and UNICEF.

In 2008, the INFS organized a nutrition survey through its staff working to send relief to regions stricken by the Wenchuan Earthquake, which occurred on May 12, 2008. The earthquake had ruined large regions in the three provinces of Sichuan, Shanxi, and Gansu. More than 60,000 people died in the disaster. The data suggested that urgent intervention was needed in the region as the rates of wasting and anemia reached more than 9% and 40%, respectively, while the rates were less than 3% and 25%, before the earthquake. Madam Chen and other nutrition experts appealed to the MOH to take action and provide YYB as an intervention tool or earthquake aid project for infants 6–24 months of age. Under the leadership of the MOH, the INFS was responsible for the implementation of the 'Infants Nutrition Intervention Project in Wenchuan Earthquake Regions'. The INFS started the intervention with YYB in three counties in earthquake regions in the Sichuan Province 2 months after the earthquake. The survey data showed that the anemia rate decreased dramatically [4, 5].

The national standard of complementary food supplements was proven by the MOH after a strict procedure of evaluation in December, 2009, in which YYB is listed as a category of high-protein food based on micronutrient-enriched products. The micronutrient density of YYB is higher than in other formula food, while the high-protein content is different from micronutrient powders and other dietary nutrient supplements (table 1). The establishment of the YYB standard promoted the development of the YYB project since this brand-new product would not be permitted on the market, which was obviously a huge obstacle. It was considered a breakthrough in terms of infant nutrition products.

Table 2. Projects implementing YYB or similar products in poor rural regions in China [3]

Projects	Regions	Departments involved and partners	Organizers/ funding agencies	Duration
Infant nutrition intervention in the Gansu province with YYB	Counties of Tianzhu, Jingning, Qingshui, Dingxi, and Jingtai	ILSI China, Gansu CDC, and Nestlé	ILSI/ILSI	2001–2003
YYB market promotion research	Counties of Changzi and Huguan Shanxi Province	FFO, CPI, MCH of the counties Qingdao Biomate Company	MOH/GAIN	5/2008–12/2009
Infant feeding and nutrition intervention in the Mei County	Mei County Shaanxi province	ILSI China, FFO, and CPI	UNICEF/UNICEF	8/2008–12/2009
Fortification of complementary food in infants	Counties of Yuzhong and Yongjing	FFO	UNICEF/UNICEF	5/2009–12/2009
Nutrition supplements in four western provinces	4 counties in Inner Mongolia, 3 counties in Qinghai Province, 3 counties in Guizhou Province, and 3 counties in Guangxi Province	Department and Health Center for Women and Children	MOH/ Heiz Company	10/2008–10/2011
Infant nutrition intervention with YYB in Wenchuan Earthquake rural regions	Counties of Beichuan, Mao, and Li	FFO, DOH, and MCH in the counties, Public Health College of Sichuan University Qingdao Biaomate Company	MOH/UNICEF, GAIN, ILSI, and Biaomate Company	9/2008–3/2009
Research to improve children nutrition deficiency in poor rural regions	12 counties in 6 provinces	INFS, local CDC, DSM, Beijing Longevity Vita company	Ministry of Science and Technology	2009–2010
Social justice – development of IYCN in poor regions	Ledu County, Qinghai; Xundian County, Yunnan	CDRF, local government, ILSI, FFO, and DSM	CDRF/CDRF	2009–2012
Infant nutrition intervention in Wenchuan Earthquake rural regions	5 counties in Sichuan, 2 counties in Shaanxi, and 1 county in Gansu	INFS, local CDC, and MCH Biaomate Company	MOH/UNICEF, and US CDC	5/2010–12/2011
Millennium project	Zhengan County, Guizhou; Zhenan County, Shaanxi; Wuding County, Yunnan	INFS, local CDC Biomate Company	MOH/UNICEF	2010–2011

Table 2. Continued

Projects	Regions	Departments involved and partners	Organizers/ funding agencies	Duration
Infant feeding and nutrition improvement	Regions in 12 provinces	Subbranch of children health, Society of Chinese Preventive Medicine, CPI Tiantianai Company	MOH/Tiantianai Company	2010–2012
YYB intervention in China Plan project regions	6 counties, Shaanxi; 1 county, Ningxia; 2 counties, Yunnan	China Plan	China Plan/ China Plan	2011–2012
Infant nutrition intervention in Zhouqu	Zhouqu County, Gansu	INFS	MOH/UNICEF	12/2011–11/2012
Eliminating infant anemia with YYB	33 counties in 11 provinces	Chinese Children Foundation, MCH of China CDC, local woman federation, and MCH	Women Federation, MOH/ Chinese Children Foundation	>12/2011
Improving children's nutrition in poor rural regions	Targeted to cover all poor counties in 22 provinces	MOH and Women Federation	Ministry of Finance	>10/2012

CPI = Capital Paediatrics Institute; MCH = Mother and Children Health Center; DOH = Department of Health of the Counties; CDRF = China Development and Research Foundation; IYCN = infants and young children nutrition.

After 2008, more than 15 national or regional intervention projects have been carried out in rural China (table 2), including nutrition interventions involving YYB in 8 counties in the Wenchuan Earthquake region. The MOH-organized work system was based on the public health department and hospitals at county, township, and village levels in three earthquake provinces. The practice was successful with this three-layer system, which fulfilled more than 90% of YYB coverage and compliance. All these YYB projects accumulated health benefit data and reinforced the social consensus that YYB could be a low-cost, effective method to improve nutrition in poor rural regions in China. Therefore, the MOH launched a project aiming to improve child nutrition in poor regions on October 12, 2012.

Nutrition Effects of YYB

Wang Yuying, Madam Chen, and others reported the results of YYB in an intervention study in the Gansu Province in 2004, 2006, and 2007, which suggested that the YYB-treated group had lower anemia rates, higher length-for-age and weight-for-age z-scores, as well as better cognitive scores [6–8]. In 5 poor counties of the Gansu Province, 1,478 children aged 4–12 months were enrolled and randomized into two groups. In addition to the usual home-made complementary food, all the children were fed 1 sachet of either formula I (soy bean powder enriched with vitamin D, vitamin B2, calcium, iron and zinc) or formula II per day per person, which contained either soy bean powder or rice powder (not enriched, but contained same amount of energy as formula I); a high dose of vitamin A was administered to both groups at 6-month intervals. Weight and height, hemoglobin level in the finger, and the development quotient were assessed every 3 months until 24 months of age. The study proved that application of YYB as home fortification of regular complementary feeding in poor rural regions of China may be feasible. The Gansu study suggested that YYB had four effects: it reduced stunting, underweight, and the rate of anemia, and improved cognitive performance.

Zhang et al. [9] systematically reviewed the studies of different YYB projects. Medline, PubMed, Cochrane Library, CNKI, and other sources of nutrition and health information were searched with the predetermined key words. The quality of the reports obtained was evaluated using the criteria established in this study. RevMan 5.3 was used in the meta-analysis. Thirteen groups of qualified data from 9 YYB intervention studies were used. The results showed that YYB significantly increased the level of hemoglobin (MD = 0.94, 95% CI 0.94–1.15, $p < 0.01$) and the weight-for-height z-score (MD = 0.42, 95% CI 0.19–0.65, $p < 0.01$), and reduced the prevalence of anemia (RR = 0.34, 95% CI 0.25–0.46, $p < 0.01$). Additionally, the YYB intervention groups also showed a lower prevalence of underweight (RR = 0. 53, 95% CI 0.32–0.88, $p < 0.05$). As a complementary food supplement for infants, YYB improved the nutritional status of infants and young children and increased hemoglobin levels, and decreased the rates of anemia and wasting. Observational data strongly supported the effect YYB on hemoglobin levels and anemia prevalence [10].

Improving Children's Nutrition in Poor Regions

In 2012, the MOH initialed the project 'Improving Children's Nutrition in Poor Regions' targeted at all infants 6–24 months of age in poor rural counties to integrate YYB in complementary feeding combined with information on nutritional knowledge to the guardians, and 100 million CNY were invested to purchase YYB products through bidding systems in YYB-covered provinces. Infants from 6 to 24 months of age in 100 poor counties were given YYB. Nutritional knowledge and improved complementary feeding were communicated by campaigns, post, and brochures, as well as doctor consultants and female federal employees. In 2014, the fund increased to 300 million, and 300 counties were covered. In 2015, the fund amounted to 500 million, and 341 counties were covered. It is expected that coverage will extend to all the 834 poor counties mainly located in west and middle regions. The Chinese government has invested 900 million CNY to purchase YYB products and distribute them to families in 341 poor counties covering more than 4 million infants.

Monitoring and evaluation conducted by the Chinese CDC in 1,800 infants and their guardians from 6 counties in the Shanxi, Yunnan, and Hubei Provinces evidenced that prevalence rates significantly dropped: anemia from 32.9 to 26.0%, stunting from 10.1 to 8.4%, diarrhea from 14.2 to 9.4%, costs for clinic payment from 98.8 to 74.4 CNY, and nutritional knowledge of guardians increased from 29.6 to 38.5% after 1 year; the project lasted from March 2013 to March 2014. The duration of consumption is 7.2 months, coverage of YYB is 85.9%, and utilization of YYB is 52.0%. The project planned to invest 500 million CNY in 2015 to enlarge the coverage to 341 counties involving 142 million infants (table 2).

The coverage of YYB will be enlarged to all the 834 poor counties in China in the future. Better nutrition in children will improve their health status, and in the long run, it will help people living in poor counties to recover from poverty and the heavy burden of malnutrition and (associated) diseases. According to the national nutrition strategy, infants and young children or early life within the first 1,000 days are one of the priorities. The YYB studies presented indicate the effectiveness of this fortification method, and YYB might also be beneficial for malnourished infants in other developing countries to improve nutrition and health. To strengthen the scientific observations and research on YYB, further studies aiming to improve the formula, randomized controlled trials, and cost-benefit analyses are warranted, for example. The working system for YYB project implementation should also be studied in terms of sustainability.

Disclosure Statement

The authors declare no conflict of interest in this study; in particular, they are not directly or indirectly affiliated to any profit-making units related to the YYB intervention. This study was supported by UNICEF. The author is deeply indebted to Sun Jing, Su Yingchang, Huang Jian and other colleagues for their effort to YYB evaluation.

References

1 Chang S, Wu H, Jia F, et al: Analysis on the changes of nutritional status in China – anemia status of children under 5 in China (in Chinese). Wei Sheng Yan Jiu 2007;36:210–212.
2 Chang S, Chen CM, He W, et al: Analysis on the changes of nutritional status in China-the improvement of complementary feeding among Chinese infants and young children (in Chinese). Wei Sheng Yan Jiu 2007;36:207–209.
3 Huo J, Sun J, Huang J, et al: Technical Guidelines of Complementary Food Supplements. Beijing, Chinese Standard Press, 2013.
4 Wang L, Huo J, Sun J, et al: Nutrition effectiveness of infants and young children aged 6 to 23 months by Ying Yang Bao in the Lixian County affected by the Wenchuan Earthquake in the Sichuan Province (in Chinese). Wei Sheng Yan Jiu 2011;40:61–64.
5 Sun J, Huo J, Zhao L, et al: The nutritional status of young children and feeding practices two years after the Wenchuan Earthquake in the worst-affected areas in China. Asia Pac J Clin Nutr 2013;22:100–108.
6 Wang Y, Chen C, Jia M, et al: Effect of complementary food supplements on anemia in infants and young children (in Chinese). Wei Sheng Yan Jiu 2004;33:334–336.
7 Wang Y, Chen C, Wang F, et al: Effects of nutrient-fortified complementary food supplements on the growth of infants and young children in poor rural areas in the Gansu Province (in Chinese). Wei Sheng Yan Jiu 2007;36:78–81.
8 Chen C, Wang Y, Chang S: Effect of in-home fortification of complementary feeding on intellectual development of Chinese children. Biomed Environ Sci 2010;23:83–91.
9 Zhang QN, Sun J, Jia XD, Huo JS: Meta-analysis of the nutrition intervention effect of Ying Yang Bao on infants and young children in China (in Chinese). Wei Sheng Yan Jiu 2015;44:970–977.
10 Huo JS, Sun J, Fang Z, et al: Effect of home-based complementary food fortification on prevalence of anemia among infants and young children aged 6 to 23 months in poor rural regions of China. Food Nutr Bull 2015;36:405–414.

Black RE, Makrides M, Ong KK (eds): Complementary Feeding: Building the Foundations for a Healthy Life. Nestlé Nutr Inst Workshop Ser, vol 87, pp 139–140, (DOI: 10.1159/000448976)
Nestec Ltd., Vevey/S. Karger AG., Basel, © 2017

Summary of Complementary Feeding Interventions in LMIC

The second session of the workshop focused on important aspects of complementary feeding, generally considered to be the addition of foods during ages 6–23 months when children are continuing to receive breast milk. The first speaker, *Robert E. Black*, described the faltering of growth compared to the World Health Organization (WHO) growth standards that happens in this critical period, and how this has lasting adverse effects on stunted growth and development. He also put the dietary gaps in the broader context of other determinants of poor growth, including maternal factors leading to fetal growth restriction and premature delivery, infectious diseases, such as diarrhea, and possibly heavy exposure of the intestine to pathogenic microbes leading to environmental enteropathy.

Marie T. Ruel provided a review for the indicators proposed by the WHO to assess the adequacy of complementary feeding practices. These indicators have been widely used for population level assessments with data collected in national or subnational surveys. They are simple and practical indicators of the four dimensions of complementary feeding: timing of introduction, dietary diversity, meal frequency, and intake of iron-rich foods. A number of limitations were also discussed which indicated the need for more validation, reduction of measurement errors, and better ways to assess feeding practices in the critical and rapidly changing period of the second half of infancy.

Rebecca Heidkamp followed with a presentation of the evidence for effects of complementary feeding interventions on the growth of infants and young children. Three recent systematic reviews suggest statistically significant effects of a modest size on weight and length gain from nutrition education in food-secure populations and from provision of food supplementation, including food-insecure populations. Recognizing the determinants of poor growth in addition to improved diets, it is important to consider the effects of other interventions, such as improved water, sanitation, hygiene, and food safety along with nutritional interventions if larger benefits are to be expected.

Innovative studies that developed and evaluated the effects of ready-to-use complementary foods using local ingredients in Bangladesh were presented by *Tahmeed Ahmed*. Community trials demonstrated benefits for linear growth of rice-lentil, chickpea, and Plumpy-doz complementary foods, compared to the usual diet of children 6–18 months old. Ready-to-use complementary food can be used to reduce stunting in children living in conditions of food insecurity.

Lynnette M. Neufeld provided a review of evidence on fortified commercial complementary foods and home fortification. Both generally provide the daily intake of vitamins and minerals recommended by the WHO. Home fortification has been with micronutrient powders, usually in a single-dose sachet, or small-quantity lipid-based nutrient supplements. While these have resulted in some improvement in the micronutrient status, especially iron, their effects on growth have been limited and variable. She also discussed aspects of product development, demand creation, and implementation research that are needed to design and conduct programs that have beneficial effects on the nutritional status.

Finally, *Junsheng Huo* presented how soy bean powder-based complementary food, Ying Yang Bao, was developed and used to improve nutrition of young children in poor rural areas of China. Analysis of the extensive testing of the product in China showed that its consumption decreased anemia and increased weight gain. The use of Ying Yang Bao is being scaled up by the government to cover all 6- to 24-month-old infants in poor rural countries along with nutrition education. Four million infants have already been included in the program.

Robert E. Black

Black RE, Makrides M, Ong KK (eds): Complementary Feeding: Building the Foundations for a Healthy Life. Nestlé Nutr Inst Workshop Ser, vol 87, pp 141–151, (DOI: 10.1159/000448964)
Nestec Ltd., Vevey/S. Karger AG., Basel, © 2017

Healthy Growth and Development

Ken K. Ong

MRC Epidemiology Unit, Institute of Metabolic Science, University of Cambridge, Cambridge, UK

Abstract

Observational and experimental studies indicate a remarkably consistent association between rapid growth and weight gain during infancy and higher risks for obesity in later childhood and adult life. This association appears to be equally relevant to breastfed and formula milk-fed infants, and infants small for gestational age and with normal birth weight. The type of infant milk feeding, energy intake, and milk nutrient composition are important determinants of infant growth and weight gain. There is also accumulating evidence that genetic factors related to adult obesity susceptibility act in the central nervous system to regulate intrinsic levels of infant appetite and satiety, and they impact on infant dietary behaviors to influence growth and weight gain. These genetic factors indicate an early life trajectory to later obesity that starts with rapid infancy gains in weight, length, and fat and lean mass, before the subsequent emergence of high BMI and adiposity. Better understanding of the anthropometric, metabolic and behavioral correlates of this trajectory will help to enable early-life prediction and preventive strategies against obesity and related metabolic disorders.

Rapid Infancy Weight Gain and Later Obesity Risk

Observational studies over the last 20 years have described the remarkably consistent association between rapid growth and weight gain during infancy and higher risks for obesity in later childhood and adult life. In the most recent review, 45/46 studies reported a positive association between higher infancy weight or weight gain and later childhood overweight [1]. Such studies have been reported in settings across the world and are supported by experimental evidence from the long-term follow-up of randomized controlled trials of newborn feeding regimens in preterm and small-for-gestational-age infants [2]. The likely relevance to the rising global obesity burden is indicated by secular trends towards faster infancy weight gain and rising prevalence of overweight and obesity in young children [3].

While the overall association between rapid infancy weight gain and later obesity had been established even 10 years ago, in order to inform prediction and preventive strategies, more detailed understanding was needed on the shape of the association and its applicability to population groups. To address these questions, a meta-analysis of pooled individual level data was performed across 10 studies and involving nearly 45,000 participants [4]. This showed a continuous influence of rising infancy weight gain on the risk of childhood obesity, as well as a substantially higher risk in those infants who crossed upwards through >2 weight centile bands (>1.33 z-scores). Those findings indicate the potential benefits for both population-wide and also targeted high-risk preventive strategies starting in early life. Furthermore, that pooled meta-analysis showed that the relevance of rapid infant weight gain for childhood obesity appears to be similar in breastfed and formula-fed infants, and in small-for-gestational-age and normal-birth weight infants [4].

In addition to higher childhood BMI and obesity risk, rapid infancy weight gain appears also to promote higher levels of central adiposity, insulin resistance, childhood adrenal and gonadal sex hormones, and earlier pubertal timing [5]. In turn, earlier pubertal timing in both males and females has been robustly associated with higher risks for type II diabetes, cardiovascular disease, various reproductive cancers, and all-cause mortality [6, 7]. Rapid infancy weight gain may therefore represent not only a faster trajectory of childhood growth and development, but also of long-term aging, health, and survival.

Feeding for Healthy Infancy Weight Gain

As we turn to consider the determinants of rapid infancy weight gain, it is important to recognize that infant feeding is the result of a complex interaction and signaling between the mother and the infant [8]. In humans as in other species, mothers recognize and respond to their infant's feeding cues. These communications may be altered by setting and type of feeding, with potential consequences for adult chronic disease risk [9]. Here, we consider separately the impact of infant feeding patterns on infancy weight gain, before describing emerging evidence for factors that are intrinsic within the infant, in particular the genetic regulation of infant feeding behavior. However, future studies are needed to study their likely interactions.

Possibly, the most established impact of infant feeding on infant growth is demonstrated by the different weight gain trajectories of breastfed and formula-fed infants. Invariably, at least among high-income countries and other socially advantaged groups, breastfed infants follow a slower trajectory of weight gain [10]. This difference underlies the rationale for the WHO 2006 Growth Standard for children aged 0–5 years, which was based on predominantly breastfed infants in high socioeconomic settings, and represents a slower more optimal trajectory of weight gain compared to previous growth references based on predominantly formula-fed Western cohorts. An assessment, performed to inform the adoption of these WHO growth charts in the UK, predicted their substantial (and likely beneficial) impact on the classification of more young children as being in overweight and obese categories, and far fewer infants and young children as having underweight or poor infancy weight gain [11].

The relevance for later obesity of the slower weight gain trajectory of breastfed infants has been hotly debated. Those that champion the null hypothesis often base their judgment on the ineffectiveness on childhood BMI of a large experimental trial of breastfeeding promotion, the PROBIT study in Belarus [12]. However, in that setting, breastfeeding promotion reduced the high prevalence of gastrointestinal and respiratory infections, and promoted a higher trajectory of infant weight during the first 12 months [13]. Therefore, if the protective role of breastfeeding in obesity were to act through the (infancy) Growth Acceleration hypothesis [14], the PROBIT data may not be representative of breastfeeding in more developed eras and settings.

Adoption of the WHO 2006 Growth Standard highlights the question: why do formula-fed infants grow faster than breastfed infants (at least in Western cohorts). Several possible explanations have been mooted, ranging from differences in milk nutrient composition, to diminished infant satiety cues, and even (where formula milk feeding is highly prevalent) a changed (i.e. lower) sociocultural expectation of normal infant signaling [15].

With regard to nutrient composition, evidence has accumulated that milk formulas with high-protein content promote rapid infancy weight gain. Such findings, together with improved protein quality, have contributed to significant lowering of protein contents of most formula preparations [16]. A recent observational study of the (substantially more variable) nutrient composition of human breast milk supports a positive effect of milk protein on infant weight, and also suggests a potential satiating and weight-limiting role of milk fat content [17]. Although milk intakes were not assessed in that study, fat intake at age 2 years has been independently reported to be inversely associated with adiposity at age 10 years and serum leptin concentrations at age 20 years [18].

Beyond milk nutrient composition, there appears to be a linear relationship between total energy intake and weight gain during infancy, at least among formula-fed infants [19]. A recent UK national survey demonstrated substantially higher average energy intakes in infants and young children compared to current recommendations (DNSIYC). Such observations indicate that very many infants have excessive calorie intakes. While the implication for limiting infant intakes may appear to be straightforward, effective shifting downwards of population level infant energy intakes requires a sensitive understanding of parental attitudes and aspirations for their infant's growth, which often may be higher than optimal, and may have been influenced by experiences of food insecurity [20]. Support is also needed to help parents to manage those infants with high intrinsic levels of appetite.

Studies have also variably reported an association between earlier age at the introduction of complementary feeding (solid foods) and higher risk for later obesity. In some studies, this association is seen only among formula-fed infants, while in others it is attenuated by adjustment for socioeconomic factors and infant milk feeding [1]. A recent systematic review has shed doubt on the underlying premise that early introduction of solids ('weaning') might increase later obesity by promoting a higher rate of infant weight gain [21]. While 10/15 studies observed higher infant weights in those who were weaned earlier, most of those studies with available data to test for reverse causality found that rapid infant weight gain preceded the introduction of solids. The authors concluded that, consistent with the results of two experimental trials, age at weaning appears to have neutral effects on infant growth. Rather, early age at weaning may be influenced by parental responses to a larger infant size, rapid growth and weight gain, or even higher signaling of hunger cues by the infant [21].

Infant Control of Infant Weight Gain

The concept that factors intrinsic within the infant might contribute to their level of appetite, food intake, and weight gain has long been suggested by anecdotal evidence in poorly growing but otherwise healthy infants with nonorganic 'failure to thrive'. More recently, it has been substantiated by studies of rare monogenic obesity, common genetic polymorphisms, and infant feeding behavior.

Twin studies have estimated that the heritability of BMI is high even in very young children [22]. The most recent genome-wide association study for BMI (studied in huge numbers of adults) reported 97 common genetic variants with highly robust and independent association signals [23]. While the identity of the underlying mechanisms requires much future work, there was remarkably strong enrichment of association signals located in or near genes that are expressed in the central nervous system, particularly the hypothalamus and pituitary gland, suggesting a predominantly 'central' genetic regulation of weight gain and BMI. Crucial to the topic of this review, longitudinal studies show that those common genetic variants affect weight gain during infancy and childhood, but not during adult life – rather their impact on higher attained body weight persists through adult life with adverse consequences for type II diabetes and other obesity-related metabolic disorders [24]. Notably, those genetic variants appear to act across the spectrum of infancy weight gain, being protective against 'inadequate' levels of weight gain while also predisposing to overweight and obesity [25].

Monogenic studies of severe early-onset obesity have identified rare deleterious mutations in/around a dozen genes. Those findings have delineated the potent regulation of appetite and satiety by the hypothalamus [26]. Affected children are characterized by extremely high and insatiable appetites ('hyperphagia') from infancy. A recent report described a rare mutation causing a bioinactive form of the satiety signaling hormone leptin [27]. After 4 weeks of full breastfeeding, one affected sibling developed an insatiable appetite leading to the introduction of bottle-feeding at age 5 weeks.

Within the general population, the relevance of intrinsic interindividual differences in infant appetite on infant weight gain has been shown in recent years by studies that have taken advantage of pioneering work to characterize and quantify differences in infant eating behavior in large-scale studies. Llewellyn and Wardle [28] identified distinct appetitive constructs relating to either food responsiveness (appetite) or satiety responsiveness. In their twin studies, these early-life traits showed significant heritability, and they were predictive of infant weight gain and later body size. Furthermore, both in children and in adults, such eating behavior traits have been positively related to the same common genetic variants that were identified for their highly robust associations with adult BMI and obesity risk [28]. Therefore, it appears that common genetic factors acting centrally in the brain contribute to the wide interindividual differences in levels of infant appetite, satiety, food intake, and weight gain, and they provide both epidemiological and biological links between early growth and feeding behaviors to later childhood pubertal timing and adult metabolic disease risks.

Healthy Body Composition in Infancy?

Body composition changes markedly during the first 12 months of life. Relative adiposity, indicated by percent body fat, rises markedly from birth, reaching a peak at around the age of 8 months, and then declines steadily until the age at adiposity rebound, typically around 4–7 years of age. While it may appear logical to assume that infants with higher relative adiposity may be at higher long-term risk of obesity and its metabolic consequences, the data are yet sparse. In contrast to the wealth of data on infant weight gain in relation to later childhood and adult outcomes [1], studies that have assessed body composition in infants are far more recent, and therefore we currently lack long-term follow-up of those cohorts. To date, only one very small US study of 53 term infants has assessed the relevance of fat and lean mass gains during infancy on risks for overweight in childhood at 9 years of age [29]. Each 100 g/month gain in infancy body weight or fat mass between birth to 8 months was associated with a ~5- or 8-fold higher risk of childhood overweight, respectively; however, the 95% confidence intervals were extremely wide and overlapping, and (although nonsignificant) the association with infancy lean mass gain was very similar (~5-fold).

In the absence of long-term follow-up data, informative insights may be gained by studying the patterns of association on infant body composition of those common genetic variants that have robust associations with adult BMI and obesity risk. Firstly, those studies indicate a positive influence of those obesity susceptibility variants on infant length gain as well as weight gain [25, 30]. Notably, this positive impact on infant (and childhood) stature differs from the lack of association with adult height; this may be explained by an earlier timing of pubertal development and therefore earlier cessation of childhood height gain. As a consequence, weight-for-length (i.e. BMI) changes underestimate the full impact of these genetic variants in early life. Secondly, and consistent with their positive impact on infant length gain, those obesity susceptibility variants appear to promote symmetrical gains in infancy fat and lean mass (fig. 1) [30]. Again, these observations in infancy run contrary to findings in later childhood and in adults, where predominant effects of these variants are seen on relative adiposity [23]. This unusual effect of obesity susceptibility variants on stature and lean body mass in infancy may be consistent with the unusual endocrine regulation of insulin-like growth factor-1 generation and length growth during this life period, which are largely independent of growth hormone but instead are dependent on nutrition [31].

The clinical implication of these insights is that, in an infant who demonstrates rapid weight gain, coincident rapid gains in body length and lean mass are not always reassuring regarding their long-term risk for obesity. Rather, many such infants will likely develop increasing BMI and adiposity through childhood, leading to earlier puberty timing and neutral (or even negative) effects on their adult height. It is certainly possible that infants with rapid weight gain who also deposit relatively more fat mass, and central fat, will be especially highly predisposed to obesity and its metabolic consequences. However, as yet,

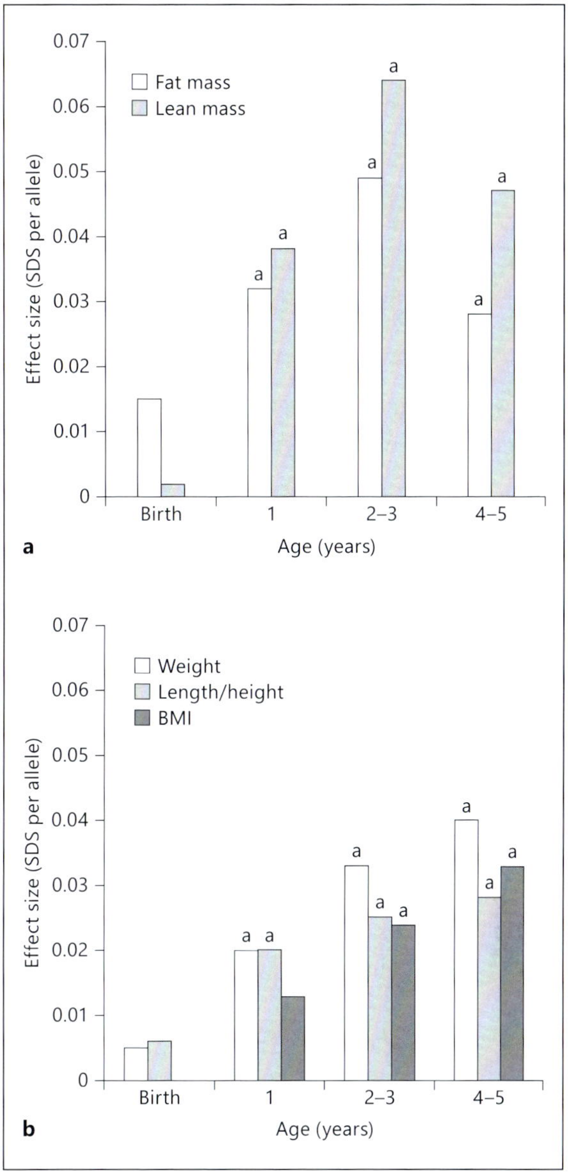

Fig. 1. Cross-sectional associations between the obesity risk allele score and early childhood body size and composition ([a] $p < 0.05$). **a** Fat and lean mass. **b** Weight, length/height, and BMI SDS. Reproduced with permission from Elks et al. [30].

the long-term relevance of those body composition changes has not been determined.

The uncertainty about the long-term health relevance of infant adiposity is further illustrated by the observation that breastfed infants initially gain more rapidly in relative adiposity than formula-fed infants. A recent systematic review identified 15 studies comprising over 1,000 infants and concluded that formula-fed infants have higher levels of fat-free mass than breastfed infants during the

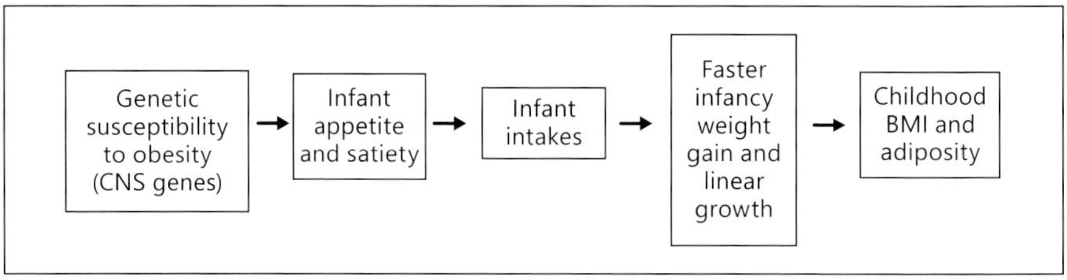

Fig. 2. Hypothesized mechanism linking adult genetic obesity susceptibility variants with infant and childhood eating behavior, dietary intakes, and growth.

first year of life; formula-fed infants also have lower fat mass and lower percent body fat at 3–6 months of age, but intriguingly this adiposity difference between groups is reversed by 12 months of age [32]. Similar to the findings of the above genetic studies [30] and studies in small-for-gestational-age infants [33], this comparison of infant milk feeding groups indicates that rapid gains in lean body mass are not necessarily protective against future obesity and that, in infants with rapid weight gain, the emergence of higher percent body fat may be a relatively late occurrence (fig. 2).

Future Perspectives

While we await longer-term follow-up studies to inform the relevance of infant body composition changes, we should ask whether we have indeed assessed the most informative and biologically relevant parameters of infant growth and associated metabolic changes. Some further possible markers are discussed below.

Healthy Body Shape

The anthropometric and body composition measures collected in infant studies usually unwittingly follow those that have been developed in studies of middle-aged and older adults. In epidemiological studies in adults, measurements are prioritized on their abilities to (i) discriminate between individuals and (ii) to predict incident disease and mortality. However, in both of these regards, their application to infants and young children may not be optimal. While weight gain in middle-aged and older adults leads to predominant accumulation of fat mass rather than lean mass, as described above, in infancy nutrition promotes length gain and fat-free mass in addition to fat mass and overall body weight [30–32]. The consequence of this scenario may be illustrated by the surprising findings of a recent comprehensive assessment of early childhood body size and shape using 3D photonic scanning. Unsupervised principal component analysis showed that in 6-year-old Brazilian children almost all traditional measures of body size and body composition cluster closely together [34]. Hence, BMI was not only strongly positively correlated with weight, waist circumference, and fat mass, but also with height, hip circumference, lean mass, and bone mass. This means that 'detailed' body composition assessment provides no further ability to discriminate between 6-year-old children than simply recording their body weight! However, three additional novel components of body shape and size were observed: the 'central-to-peripheral ratio' (positively related to torso surface area and inversely related to leg length and volume); 'height and arm lengths', and 'upper shoulder diameter' [34]. Observed differences in those novel components by sex, birth weight, socioeconomic status, and skin color suggest that they might have potential relevance to lead to disease risks.

Healthy Biomarkers

Recent technological advances in large-scale assays (requiring tiny sample volumes) now allow assessment of an infant's biology and metabolism on a systematic and unprecedented scale. Microbiome composition can be characterized using powerful next-generation sequencing of the 16s-rRNA gene – recent studies show marked differences in stool microbial community composition by infant feeding and mode of delivery [35]. Metabolomic, lipidomic, and hormone assays on infant capillary blood samples have been validated. High-resolution mass spectrometry has allowed the identification of distinct infant lipidomic profiles between breastfed and formula-fed infants, and an intermediate profile in mixed-fed infants [36].

As discussed above, the long-term relevance of these and other detailed characteristics of infant growth and metabolism are yet unknown. In the short term, research studies that aim to categorize the infant phenotypes associated with low versus high genetic obesity susceptibility might inform which infant profiles are indicative of future health.

Lastly, it should be noted that the obesity susceptibility variants appear to have far less relevance to the rapid postnatal catch-up weight gain and growth that typically occurs in infants with low birth weight or small for gestational age [30]. Rapid weight gain in these infants is still likely to be detrimental to their future metabolic health risks [4]. However, their (putative) higher levels of appetite signaling and energy intake are likely driven by other mechanisms. For example, low circulating leptin levels are suggested to link low birth weight to rapid postnatal weight gain. The application of sensitive multiplex assays in clinical research studies will allow more systematic assessments of the potential roles of circulating adipocyte- or gut-derived appetite-regulating hormones in infancy weight gain and obesity.

Acknowledgment

K.K.O. is supported by the Medical Research Council (Unit Program No. MC_UU_12015/2). He chairs the International Life Sciences Institute, Europe, Expert Advisory Group on Early Growth Velocity and Risk of Metabolic Disorders Later in Life.

Disclosure Statement

K.K.O. receives research funding from Mead Johnson Nutrition for the discovery of biomarkers for infant nutrition.

References

1 Woo Baidal JA, Locks LM, Cheng ER, et al: Risk factors for childhood obesity in the first 1,000 days: a systematic review. Am J Prev Med 2016;50:761–779.
2 Singhal A, Kennedy K, Lanigan J, et al: Nutrition in infancy and long-term risk of obesity: evidence from 2 randomized controlled trials. Am J Clin Nutr 2010;92:1133–1144.
3 Lakshman R, Elks CE, Ong KK: Childhood obesity. Circulation 2012;126:1770–1779.
4 Druet C, Stettler N, Sharp S, et al: Prediction of childhood obesity by infancy weight gain: an individual-level meta-analysis. Paediatr Perinat Epidemiol 2012;26:19–26.
5 Ong KK, Emmett P, Northstone K, et al: Infancy weight gain predicts childhood body fat and age at menarche in girls. J Clin Endocrinol Metab 2009;94:1527–1532.
6 Charalampopoulos D, McLoughlin A, Elks CE, et al: Age at menarche and risks of all-cause and cardiovascular death: a systematic review and meta-analysis. Am J Epidemiol 2014;180:29–40.
7 Day F, Elks CE, Murray AM, et al: Puberty timing associated with diabetes, cardiovascular disease and also diverse health outcomes in men and women: the UK Biobank study. Sci Rep 2015;5:11208.
8 Wells JC: Parent-offspring conflict theory, signaling of need, and weight gain in early life. Q Rev Biol 2003;78:169–202.
9 Wells JC, Yao P, Williams JE, et al: Maternal investment, life-history strategy of the offspring and adult chronic disease risk in South Asian women in the UK. Evol Med Public Health 2016;2016:133–145.
10 Dewey KG: Growth characteristics of breast-fed compared to formula-fed infants. Biol Neonate 1998;74:94–105.
11 Wright C, Lakshman R, Emmett P, et al: Implications of adopting the WHO 2006 Child Growth Standard in the UK: two prospective cohort studies. Arch Dis Child 2007;93:566–569.
12 Casazza K, Fontaine KR, Astrup A, et al: Myths, presumptions, and facts about obesity. N Engl J Med 2013;368:446–454.
13 Kramer MS, Guo T, Platt RW, et al: Breast-feeding and infant growth: biology or bias? Pediatrics 2002;110:343–347.
14 Singhal A: Does breastfeeding protect from growth acceleration and later obesity? Nestle Nutr Workshop Ser Pediatr Program 2007; 60:15–25; discussion 25–29.
15 Lauzon-Guillain B, Wijndaele K, Clark M, et al: Breastfeeding and infant temperament at age three months. PLoS One 2012;7:e29326.
16 Koletzko B, Demmelmair H, Grote V, et al: High protein intake in young children and increased weight gain and obesity risk. Am J Clin Nutr 2016;103:303–304.
17 Prentice P, Ong KK, Schoemaker MH, et al: Breast milk nutrient content and infancy growth. Acta Paediatr 2016;105:641–647.
18 Rolland-Cachera MF, Maillot M, Deheeger M, et al: Association of nutrition in early life with body fat and serum leptin at adult age. Int J Obes (Lond) 2013;37:1116–1122.
19 Ong KK, Emmett PM, Noble S, et al: Dietary energy intake at the age of 4 months predicts postnatal weight gain and childhood body mass index. Pediatrics 2006;117:e503–e508.

20 Lindsay AC, Sussner KM, Greaney ML, et al: Latina mothers' beliefs and practices related to weight status, feeding, and the development of child overweight. Public Health Nurs 2011;28:107–118.
21 Vail B, Prentice P, Dunger DB, et al: Age at weaning and infant growth: primary analysis and systematic review. J Pediatr 2015;167: 317–324.e1.
22 Elks CE, den Hoed M, Zhao JH, et al: Variability in the heritability of body mass index: a systematic review and meta-regression. Front Endocrinol (Lausanne) 2012;3:29.
23 Locke AE, Kahali B, Berndt SI, et al: Genetic studies of body mass index yield new insights for obesity biology. Nature 2015;518:197–206.
24 Hardy R, Wills AK, Wong A, et al: Life course variations in the associations between FTO and MC4R gene variants and body size. Hum Mol Genet 2010;19:545–552.
25 Elks CE, Loos RJ, Sharp SJ, et al: Genetic markers of adult obesity risk are associated with greater early infancy weight gain and growth. PLoS Med 2010;7:e1000284.
26 van der Klaauw AA, Farooqi IS: The hunger genes: pathways to obesity. Cell 2015;161: 119–132.
27 Wabitsch M, Funcke JB, von Schnurbein J, et al: Severe early-onset obesity due to bioinactive leptin caused by a p.N103K mutation in the leptin gene. J Clin Endocrinol Metab 2015;100:3227–3230.
28 Llewellyn C, Wardle J: Behavioral susceptibility to obesity: gene-environment interplay in the development of weight. Physiol Behav 2015;152:494–501.
29 Koontz MB, Gunzler DD, Presley L, et al: Longitudinal changes in infant body composition: association with childhood obesity. Pediatr Obes 2014;9:e141–e144.
30 Elks CE, Heude B, de Zegher F, et al: Associations between genetic obesity susceptibility and early postnatal fat and lean mass: an individual participant meta-analysis. JAMA Pediatr 2014;168:1122–1130.
31 Karlberg J: A biologically-oriented mathematical model (ICP) for human growth. Acta Paediatr Scand Suppl 1989;350:70–94.
32 Gale C, Logan KM, Santhakumaran S, et al: Effect of breastfeeding compared with formula feeding on infant body composition: a systematic review and meta-analysis. Am J Clin Nutr 2012;95:656–669.
33 Ibanez L, Lopez-Bermejo A, Diaz M, et al: Catch-up growth in girls born small for gestational age precedes childhood progression to high adiposity. Fertil Steril 2011;96:220–223.
34 Santos LP, Ong KK, Day F, et al: Body shape and size in 6-year old children: assessment by three-dimensional photonic scanning. Int J Obes (Lond) 2016;40:1012–1017.
35 Madan JC, Hoen AG, Lundgren SN, et al: Association of cesarean delivery and formula supplementation with the intestinal microbiome of 6-week-old infants. JAMA Pediatr 2016;170:212–219.
36 Prentice P, Koulman A, Matthews L, et al: Lipidomic analyses, breast- and formula-feeding, and growth in infants. J Pediatr 2015; 166:276–281.e276.

Black RE, Makrides M, Ong KK (eds): Complementary Feeding: Building the Foundations for a Healthy Life. Nestlé Nutr Inst Workshop Ser, vol 87, pp 153–165, (DOI: 10.1159/000448965)
Nestec Ltd., Vevey/S. Karger AG., Basel, © 2017

Responsive Feeding: Strategies to Promote Healthy Mealtime Interactions

Maureen M. Black[a] · Kristen M. Hurley[b]

[a]RTI International, Research Triangle Park, NC, and Department of Pediatrics, University of Maryland School of Medicine, Baltimore, MD, and [b]Department of International Health, Bloomberg School of Public Health, Johns Hopkins University, Baltimore, MD, USA

Abstract

Responsive feeding is a derivative of responsive parenting that has been applied to infant and young child feeding. With a theoretical basis in the reciprocal interactions between parents and children, responsive feeding is particularly relevant during complementary feeding as young children progress from an exclusively milk-based liquid diet to the family diet and self-feeding. The period of complementary feeding includes multiple developmental changes that may threaten a successful transition and lead to growth and feeding problems. In spite of high rates of global childhood underweight, stunting, overweight, and obesity, and the inclusion of responsive feeding in the World Health Organization's Global Strategy for Infant and Young Child Feeding, there have been few intervention trials of responsive feeding. The aim of this chapter is to examine how parents and young children navigate the progression in feeding, with an emphasis on complementary feeding, and to address the following topics: (1) navigating the progression of feeding development, (2) provision of responsive feeding, (3) preventing or resolving growth and feeding problems, (4) responsive feeding research, and (5) strategies to promote healthy mealtime interactions. To advance responsive feeding research and practice, clarity is needed in both measurement and intervention strategies, guided by the reciprocity between parent and child interactions inherent in the theoretical basis of responsive feeding.

Introduction

Feeding is a major developmental task in the first years of life as infants and young children progress from an exclusively liquid diet to pureed foods, and finally to the family diet. Among infants, progression in feeding is influenced by: (1) advances in digestive and oral motor skills, (2) internal regulatory cues of hunger and satiety, and (3) advances in cognitive, fine motor, and social-emotional development that facilitate interest in food, self-regulation, and self-feeding [1]. Among parents, feeding is guided by cultural and family variations in foods, favors, textures, and eating patterns; food access and availability, and perceptions of children's growth, health, appetite, and temperament. Recommendations to guide parents through the progression of feeding often focus on what and when to feed, with limited attention to feeding behavior or how to handle variability in infants' signals regarding hunger and satiety or likes and dislikes [2]. This chapter focuses on how young children and parents navigate the progression in feeding, with an emphasis on complementary feeding and the transition from milk-based liquids to the family diet and from dependence on parent feeding to self-feeding. The paper has five sections: (1) navigating the progression of feeding development, (2) provision of responsive feeding, (3) preventing or resolving growth and feeding problems, (4) responsive feeding research, and (5) strategies to promote healthy mealtime interactions.

Navigating the Progression of Feeding Development

Internal Regulatory Cues

Infants and young children signal hunger and satiety through actions such as hand sucking, leaning forward for food, opening and closing of the mouth, head turning, and crying/fussing (see hunger signal in fig. 1). Parents' perceptions of feeding signals vary by external events, such as time of day, and both maternal and infant characteristics. Feeding signals also vary in form and intensity across infants (e.g., flexed hand position may signal hunger in some infants), contributing to interpretation confusion. Parents are often (fig. 1) more responsive to hunger signals than to satiety signals [3]. Children also express their food likes and dislikes through facial expressions and signals that may be easily confused with hunger/satiety signals. As children mature and parents and children develop consistent interaction patterns, signals are easier to interpret, but are likely to change as infants transition to complementary feeding and experience new flavors and textures.

Complementary Feeding

Complementary feeding refers to the introduction of nondairy liquids, with timing based on the 'developmental maturity of the gut and neuromuscular system, growth rate, and activity level' rather than specific age guidelines [4].

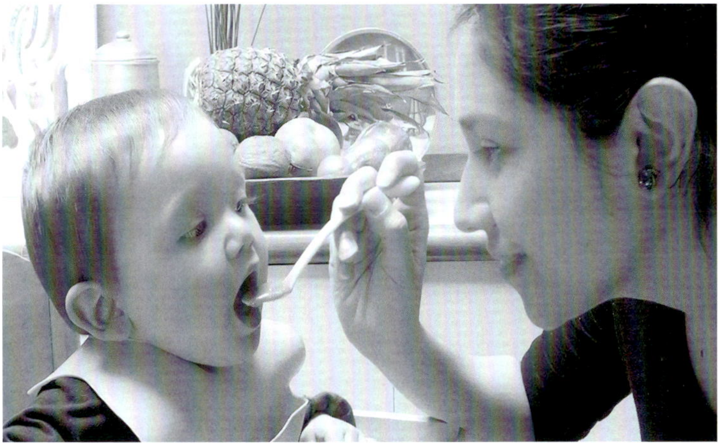

Fig. 1. Responding to an infant's signal of hunger (ProPan Complimentary Feeding Photo Contest, Pan American Health Organization/World Health Organization).

Complementary feeding typically occurs during the second 6 months of life, a period often marked by illness and weight faltering [5], the risk of micronutrient deficiencies (especially iron), and challenging hygienic practices as infants crawl on the floor and put food and objects into their mouth. During this phase, children are guided by a desire to explore their surroundings: not only what they see and hear, but also what they touch, feel, and taste. The slowdown in intake that typically occurs during the latter part of meals is influenced partially by the abatement of hunger, but also by a desire to explore the surroundings. Parents who misinterpret the slowdown as early food refusal may resort to controlling or pressuring strategies that disrupt the temporary exploration and result in mealtime stress for both parents and children.

Self-Feeding

Transitional food introduced during complementary feeding often includes purees spoon-fed by parents. Children communicate readiness to eat by signals such as opening their mouth, and the meal continues until the parent stops feeding. Self-feeding typically follows at a later developmental stage, often with small pieces of softened food and usually as a supplement to parent-fed food (fig. 2).

Baby-led weaning is a strategy that promotes self-regulation by giving infants control over feeding, rather than transitioning to parent-fed purees [6]. Baby-led weaning occurs when infants are developmentally able to pick up and bring small pieces of food to their mouth, chew, and swallow, generally

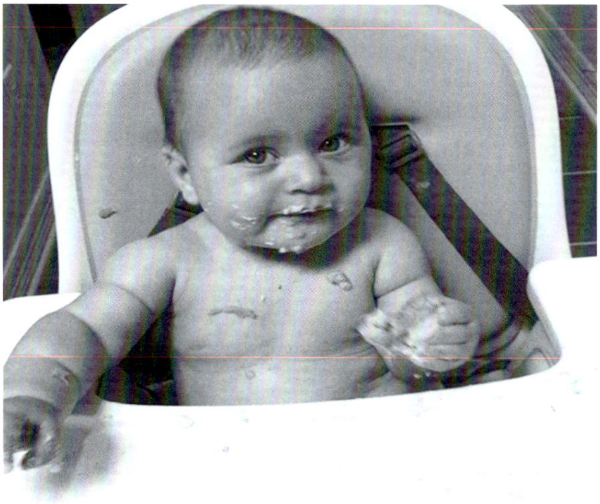

Fig. 2. Child self-feeding.

between 6 and 8 months of age (fig. 2) [7]. Although baby-led weaning is designed to occur exclusively, it is often initiated in combination with parent-fed purees.

With the exception of a recently initiated randomized trial [8], the research into baby-led weaning is generally limited to cross-sectional quantitative and qualitative studies. Advantages are thought to include a lower risk of obesity associated with self-regulatory feeding, enhanced motor development, and positive parent feeding practices [8]. Disadvantages include potential risks of choking, micronutrient deficiencies (e.g., iron and zinc), and weight faltering if the family diet is not rich in micronutrients and macronutrients. Successful baby-led weaning depends on regularly scheduled mealtimes with the family consuming and modeling a healthy diet, and offering the infant bites of appropriate size and consistency.

Four barriers to self-feeding in young children were reported by Bangladeshi mothers living in low-resource communities: (1) the time required for self-feeding, (2) the potential mess of spilled food, (3) food waste when children play with or drop food, and (4) a perception that children are unable to self-feed, leading to the possibility of hunger and associated irritability [9]. When asked about allowing children to determine how much to eat and responding to food refusal by terminating the meal, many parents expressed grave concerns about the children's ability to determine satiety and the health consequences that could result in 'sickness or death' without adequate food. Parents often reported that they had no choice other than to force-feed their children. These findings emphasize the central role that maternal beliefs, social conditions, and local customs play in parent feeding practices.

Provision of Responsive Feeding

The development of infant feeding skills is guided by parents, who are influenced by cultural, environmental, and personal factors, including food availability and resources to acquire and store food. In addition, parents are influenced by their own mental health issues, specifically depression [10], and by perceptions of their child's size, appetite, and temperament.

Responsive Parenting

Responsive feeding is often conceptualized as a derivative of responsive parenting [11]. Responsive parenting refers to the reciprocity between the parent and the child, whereby both parent and child behaviors vary in a give-and-take or serve-and-return pattern [12]. Early in life, this reciprocal process influences the emotional bonding or attachment between infants and parents that forms the basis for healthy social-emotional functioning [13]. Parenting behavior varies by parents' perceptions of their children's characteristics and behavior. For example, children perceived as temperamentally difficult are more likely to elicit harsh or restrictive parenting than children perceived as temperamentally easy or agreeable [14]. Disruptions in parent-child relationships, characterized by inconsistent and nonresponsive interactions, can undermine a child's subsequent social and emotional development [15].

Reciprocal patterns are assessed by examining both parent and child behaviors together. To be responsive, parent behavior follows child behavior, is emotionally supportive to the child, recognizes the child's behavior through a contingent action, and is related conceptually to the child's prior action (developmentally appropriate, and not passive, intrusive or controlling). Thus, parent-responsive behaviors are prompt, emotionally supportive, contingent, and developmentally appropriate [11]. Parent responsivity often occurs in the context of a supportive routine or structure whereby the child learns to expect responses that are predictable and supportive [16]. Responsive parenting is based on acknowledging the child's behavior or request, not necessarily complying with it.

Responsive parenting can be applied to the feeding context and is often characterized by feeding styles and feeding practices. Feeding styles refer to the emotional climate of the interaction, characterized by dimensions of demandingness and nurturance. *Authoritative* represents high demandingness and high nurturance, and characterizes responsive feeding. Parents communicate clear guidelines and rules, while providing nurturance and praise. *Authoritarian* represents high demandingness and low nurturance. Parents have strict rules, with little consideration of child preferences and limited nurturance. *Indulgent* represents low demandingness and high nurturance. Parents have few rules and children are permitted to eat what, where, and when they wish. *Uninvolved* represents low demandingness and low nurturance. Parents make few demands and the meals may be disorganized. Authoritarian, indulgent, and uninvolved feeding styles represent nonresponsive feeding. *Feeding practices* refer to the behaviors that parents use to organize meals and the meal structure and influence children's eating behavior.

Global Commitment to Responsive Feeding

In 2003, the World Health Organization (WHO) and UNICEF published the Global Strategy for Infant and Young Child Feeding. UNICEF had developed the Child Undernutrition Framework, which linked basic and underlying determinants to malnutrition and death. Basic determinants included political, family, and community resources. Underlying determinants included insufficient household food, insufficient health services, unhealthy environment, and poor child care practices. Responsive feeding, originally conceptualized as active feeding, in contrast to passive feeding, was one of twelve essential family care practices proposed by UNICEF.

The inclusion of care practices in the Framework led to the development of policies and publications that promoted responsive feeding [17]. Guidelines were developed to encourage parents to read children's signals of hunger and satiety, to promote self-feeding, to avoid forcing or pressuring children, and to make meals occasions for pleasant social interactions. However, there were few recommendations on strategies to prevent or handle common feeding problems, such as food refusal, and limited attention was devoted to developmental changes in children's signals and feeding behavior as they approach toddlerhood, including self-feeding, autonomy, and self-regulation.

Principles of responsive feeding have been incorporated into another WHO/UNICEF initiative, Care for Child Development [18]. Care for Child Development is an intervention package based on principles of responsive parenting, operationalized through play and communication, and designed to be implemented by community health workers [18].

Growth and Feeding Problems

Growth

Early growth is often regarded as a marker of young children's well-being. Based on longitudinal growth data for children under 5 years of age from the WHO Multicentre Growth Reference Study, growth standards have been established by WHO and UNICEF and adopted by at least 125 countries throughout the world

[19]. Using uniform standards for measuring children's weight and length [20], rates of underweight, stunting, overweight, and obesity are reported through national surveys and used as global indicators of children's growth problems. When children's growth deviates from the expected trajectories, as occurs with both underweight and overweight, attention is often directed to feeding.

Feeding

Feeding problems occur among up to 50% of typically developing infants and toddlers throughout the world, and frequently include food refusal, food selectivity (pickiness), or disruptive mealtime behavior [21, 22]. For instance, a study of toddlers in Bangladesh found relatively high rates of food refusal (mean of 6–7/meal), with fewer than 20% of mouthfuls self-fed [23]. In many cases, feeding problems represent typical toddler development of neophobia (hesitancy to try new foods) or autonomy (food refusal and desire for independence). Food refusal can be confusing to parents because it may be unclear whether children are signaling satiety, requesting an alternative, or exhibiting a behavioral problem. Early feeding problems are often transient and resolve over time, particularly when parents are sensitive to their child's signals of satiety and emerging autonomy and adhere to regularly scheduled mealtime routines. However, when feeding problems are associated with family stress [24], they can result in weight-related problems (either underweight or overweight), nutrition-related health conditions, and long-term behavioral problems [25].

Toddler feeding problems can increase in severity when parents misinterpret their toddler's signals or mismanage the situation by not providing a mealtime routine, relying on low-nutrient-dense foods, or attempting to force their toddler to eat. Education on strategies to promote healthy child feeding behavior is often provided through information sharing strategies, such as leaflets. However, evidence has shown that to be effective, education should be provided before feeding problems occur, should include parent social support, and should provide opportunities to simulate the recommended practices [26]. A recent intervention in Australia that included an 8-session group-based, behavioral intervention was effective in reducing feeding problems among typically developing children, as measured by parent report and direct observation [27].

Responsive Feeding Research

Most research related to responsive feeding has been cross-sectional and conducted from a unidirectional perspective: how parent feeding styles and practices impact child behavior and growth. More recently, longitudinal and intervention trials have focused on the interactive nature of feeding whereby parents and children respond to one another.

Aboud et al. [28] have conducted several trials related to responsive feeding in Bangladesh. In one, they found that infants (12–24 months of age) of mothers in the responsive feeding intervention had greater weight gain and demonstrated more self-feeding than infants of mothers who received a general nutrition intervention, with no difference in observed maternal feeding behavior. A second trial that demonstrated and coached parents of children aged 8–20 months to adopt responsive feeding behaviors was successful in increasing child hand washing, self-feeding, and maternal verbal responsivity, with no difference in weight gain [23]. A third trial found beneficial effects of a responsive feeding intervention on maternal responsiveness, with beneficial effects on child growth among the group that included both maternal responsiveness and micronutrient fortification [29].

A clinical intervention among young children with weight faltering in the United States found that a responsive feeding intervention with video-recorded mealtimes and interaction coaching was associated with weight gain [30]. Weight recovery over 6 months was greater among children under versus above 24 months of age and among children with multiple child and household risk factors.

A recent review focused on interventions to prevent overweight among infants identified 4 of 24 behavioral interventions that included elements of responsive feeding, primarily strategies to recognize and respond to infant signals [31]. All were conducted in high-income countries. In the NOURISH trial, intervention was conducted in infancy with follow-up through 5 years, and intervention mothers reported increased use of instrumental feeding practices, with a nonsignificant trend for lower child BMI z-scores [32]. In a second trial involving low-income, African-American, adolescent mothers, intervention group participants were more likely to adhere to the American Academy of Pediatrics guidelines on infant feeding than the control group [33]. The third trial involved a behavioral intervention with information about satiety signals and milk preparation delivered to formula-feeding parents in the Special Supplemental Nutrition Program for Women, Infants and Children [34]. Intervention group participants had better knowledge about infant feeding, but their infants had greater growth, compared to the control group. Finally, the SLIMTIME (US Sleeping and Intake Methods Taught to Infants and Mothers Early in Life) intervention, delivered to first-time mothers who intended to breastfeed, included responsive feeding messages rather than dietary advice [35]. Infants of intervention group participants had a significantly slower rate of weight gain than the control group.

These studies illustrate the beneficial effects that can be derived from responsive feeding interventions during infancy. Although there is evidence that responsive feeding may be protective against both underweight and overweight

[36], the findings have been mixed, with stronger effects on changes in feeding behavior than in weight [31]. Longer follow-up periods may be necessary to gain a better understanding as to how responsive feeding impacts the development of subsequent eating behaviors and growth patterns.

Strategies to Promote Healthy Mealtime Interactions

Strategies to promote healthy mealtime interactions include (table 1): (1) assurance that the feeding context is pleasant with few distractions, that the child is seated comfortably ideally facing others, that expectations are communicated clearly, and that foods are healthy, tasty, developmentally appropriate, and offered on a predictable schedule so the child is likely to be hungry; (2) an emotional climate whereby the parent models eating, offers encouragement as needed, and attends to the child's signals of hunger and satiety, and (3) the parent responds to the child in a prompt, emotionally supportive, contingent, and developmentally appropriate manner. With parent patience and adherence to a regular mealtime routine (2–3 h between meals, 20–30 min/meal), and limited availability and access to low-nutrient-dense foods, transient feeding problems often resolve. Findings from responsive parenting research suggest that responsive feeding promotes children's attentiveness and interest in feeding, attention to their internal signals of hunger and satiety, ability to communicate needs to their parent with distinct and meaningful signals, and successful progression to independent feeding.

Responsive feeding acknowledges children's feelings and allows them to determine how much they eat, while the parent decides what is offered and when [37]. Embedded within the domain of responsive parenting, responsive feeding emphasizes the interactive nature of feeding, whereby parents set guidelines, with their reactions gaged to the signals they read from their children, resulting in a respectful give and take around feeding.

Investigators have identified several feeding strategies that increase the likelihood of children eating, including using positive verbal encouragement versus no verbalization or mechanical verbalizations (e.g., 'eat eat') [38], and modeling healthy eating, rather than telling children to eat. Positioning children to face parents promotes modeling and enables parents to read children's signals and monitor their behavior. When toddlers are fed while seated on their parent's lap, as they are in many parts of the world, parents are unable to model eating and may have difficulty seeing the child's face, interfering with their ability to recognize, interpret, and respond to the child's signals.

Studies of responsive feeding lead to future research recommendations. Methodological advances and consistency in measurement would advance the

Table 1. Strategies to promote healthy mealtime interaction

Domain	Description	Positive Strategies
Navigating the progression of the feeding development	1 Recognizing and responding to a child's signals of hunger and satiety 2 Providing healthy and developmentally appropriate complementary food 3 Promoting self-feeding	1 Assure Feeding context is pleasant with few distractions Child is seated comfortably facing others Expectations are communicated clearly 2 Offer Tasty, healthy, developmentally appropriate foods 3 Provide Emotional climate with parent modeling eating Encourage as needed Opportunity to self-feed with developmentally appropriate food
Providing responsive feeding context	1 Responsive (authoritative) feeding style 2 Predictable feeding practices (behaviors that parents use to organize meals and the meal structure)	1 Provide food In a prompt, emotionally supportive, contingent, and developmentally appropriate manner 2 Offer foods On a predictable schedule so the child is likely to be hungry
Prevent/resolve growth and feeding problems	1 Food refusal, food selectivity (pickiness), or disruptive mealtime behavior, resulting in growth, nutrition and behaviors problems	1 Provide Patience and adherence to a regular mealtime routine (2–3 h between meals, 20–30 min/meal) resolve transient feeding problems

field [39]. The majority of studies have employed a cross-sectional design, thereby limiting examination of causal pathways. Naturalistic observations of feeding are needed in low- and middle-income countries, together with an understanding of the decisions behind feeding practices, followed by intervention trials. Multiple outcomes have been measured. Investigators could examine how responsive feeding relates to feeding behavior and weight, and whether relations differ between the two outcomes. Finally, investigators could examine the continuity/discontinuity of responsive feeding across development stages.

Conclusions

Responsive feeding, based on the underlying theory of responsive parenting, focuses on parent-child interactions during feeding episodes. As applied to complementary feeding, responsive feeding broadens the conceptual framework beyond the parent to include the contributions of the child and context.

Complementary feeding typically begins during the second 6 months of life, a period of rapid growth that includes multiple developmental changes, along with nutritional and health risks. As infants and young children strive for autonomy, neophobia and food refusal are common problems that can interfere with successful transition. Responsive feeding provides the guidelines that enable parents to avoid and manage transitional feeding problems and promote the successful transition to the family meal and self-feeding.

Although advances have been made in promoting complementary feeding and reducing feeding problems, underweight, stunting, overweight, and obesity remain major public health problems and present threats to children's long-term health, development, and well-being. Incorporating responsive feeding into nutritional interventions may be an effective strategy to promote healthy feeding behaviors early in life and to avoid the negative and life-long consequences associated with growth and feeding problems.

Disclosure Statement

M.M.B. and K.M.H. have no disclosures.

References

1 Birch LL: Learning to eat: behavioral and psychological aspects; in Fewtrell MS, Haschke F, Prescott SL (eds): Preventive Aspects of Early Nutrition. Nestlé Nutr Inst Workshop Ser. Basel, Karger, 2016, vol 85, pp 125–134.

2 Schwartz C, Scholtens PA, Lalanne A, et al: Development of healthy eating habits early in life. Review of recent evidence and selected guidelines. Appetite 2011;57:796–807.

3 Hodges EA, Johnson SL, Hughes SO, et al: Development of the responsiveness to child feeding cues scale. Appetite 2013;65:210–219.

4 Kleinman RE, Coletta FA: Historical overview of transitional feeding recommendations and vegetable feeding practices for infants and young children. Nutr Today 2016; 51:7–13.

5 Shrimpton R, Victora CG, de Onis M, et al: Worldwide timing of growth faltering: implications for nutritional interventions. Pediatrics 2001;107:E75.

6 Rapley G: Baby-led weaning: a developmental approach to the introduction of complementary foods; in Moran VH (ed): Maternal and Infant Nutrition and Nurture: Controversies and Challenges. London, Quay Books, 2013, pp 261–283.

7 Wright CM, Cameron K, Tsiaka M, et al: Is baby-led weaning feasible? When do babies first reach out for and eat finger foods? Matern Child Nutr 2011;7:27–33.

8 Daniels L, Heath A-LM, Williams SM, et al: Baby-Led Introduction to SolidS (BLISS) study: a randomised controlled trial of a baby-led approach to complementary feeding. BMC Pediatr 2015;15:179.

9 Affleck W, Pelto G: Caregivers' responses to an intervention to improve young child feeding behaviors in rural Bangladesh: a mixed method study of the facilitators and barriers to change. Soc Sci Med 2012;75:651–658.

10 Hurley KM, Black MM, Papas MA, et al: Maternal symptoms of stress, depression, and anxiety are related to nonresponsive feeding styles in a statewide sample of WIC participants. J Nutr 2008;138:799–805.
11 Black MM, Aboud FE: Responsive feeding is embedded in a theoretical framework of responsive parenting. J Nutr 2011;141:490–494.
12 Sameroff AJ (ed): The Transactional Model of Development: How Children and Contexts Shape Each Other, ed 1. Washington, American Psychological Association, 2009.
13 Ainsworth M, Blehar M, Waters E, Wall S: Patterns of Attachment: A Psychological Study of the Strange Situation. Hillsdale, Erlbaum, 1978.
14 Bergmeier H, Skouteris H, Horwood S, et al: Associations between child temperament, maternal feeding practices and child body mass index during the preschool years: a systematic review of the literature. Obes Rev 2014;15:9–18.
15 Kochanska G, Woodard J, Kim S, et al: Positive socialization mechanisms in secure and insecure parent-child dyads: two longitudinal studies. J Child Psychol Psychiatry 2010;51: 998–1009.
16 McGowan L, Cooke LJ, Gardner B, et al: Healthy feeding habits: efficacy results from a cluster-randomized, controlled exploratory trial of a novel, habit-based intervention with parents. Am J Clin Nutr 2013;98:769–777.
17 WHO, UNICEF: Global Strategy for Infant and Young Child Feeding. Geneva, World Health Organization, 2003.
18 UNICEF: Care for Child Development Package. 2012.
19 de Onis M, Onyango A, Borghi E, et al: Worldwide implementation of the WHO Child Growth Standards. Public Health Nutr 2012;15:1603–1610.
20 Ng M, Fleming T, Robinson M, et al: Global, regional, and national prevalence of overweight and obesity in children and adults during 1980–2013: a systematic analysis for the Global Burden of Disease Study 2013. Lancet 2014;384:766–781.
21 Lewinsohn PM, Holm-Denoma JM, Gau JM, et al: Problematic eating and feeding behaviors of 36-month-old children. Int J Eat Disord 2005;38:208–219.
22 Skinner JD, Carruth BR, Houck K, et al: Mealtime communication patterns of infants from 2 to 24 months of age. J Nutr Educ Behav 1998;30:8–16.
23 Aboud FE, Shafique S, Akhter S: A responsive feeding intervention increases children's self-feeding and maternal responsiveness but not weight gain. J Nutr 2009;139:1738–1743.
24 Sanders MR, Patel RK, Le Grice B, et al: Children with persistent feeding difficulties: an observational analysis of the feeding interactions of problem and non-problem eaters. Health Psychol 1993;12:64–73.
25 Nicklas TA, Hayes D; American Dietetic Association: Position of the American Dietetic Association: nutrition guidance for healthy children ages 2 to 11 years. J Am Diet Assoc 2008;108:1038–1044, 1046–1047.
26 Mitchell GL, Farrow C, Haycraft E, et al: Parental influences on children's eating behaviour and characteristics of successful parent-focussed interventions. Appetite 2013;60: 85–94.
27 Adamson M, Morawska A, Sanders MR: Childhood feeding difficulties: a randomized controlled trial of a group-based parenting intervention. J Dev Behav Pediatr 2013;34: 293–302.
28 Aboud FE, Moore AC, Akhter S: Effectiveness of a community-based responsive feeding programme in rural Bangladesh: a cluster randomized field trial. Matern Child Nutr 2008;4:275–286.
29 Aboud FE, Akhter S: A cluster-randomized evaluation of a responsive stimulation and feeding intervention in Bangladesh. Pediatrics 2011;127:e1191–e1197.
30 Black MM, Tilton N, Bento S, et al: Recovery in young children with weight faltering: child and household risk factors. J Pediatr 2016; 170:301–306.
31 Redsell SA, Edmonds B, Swift JA, et al: Systematic review of randomised controlled trials of interventions that aim to reduce the risk, either directly or indirectly, of overweight and obesity in infancy and early childhood. Matern Child Nutr 2016;12:24–38.
32 Daniels LA, Mallan KM, Nicholson JM, et al: An early feeding practices intervention for obesity prevention. Pediatrics 2015;136:e40–e49.

33 Black MM, Siegel E, Abel Y, et al: Home and videotape intervention delays early complementary feeding among adolescent mothers. Pediatrics 2001;107:E67.
34 Kavanagh KF, Cohen RJ, Heinig MJ, et al: Educational intervention to modify bottle-feeding behaviors among formula-feeding mothers in the WIC program: impact on infant formula intake and weight gain. J Nutr Educ Behav 2008;40:244–250.
35 Paul IM, Savage JS, Anzman SL, et al: Preventing obesity during infancy: a pilot study. Obesity 2011;19:353–361.
36 DiSantis KI, Hodges EA, Johnson SL, et al: The role of responsive feeding in overweight during infancy and toddlerhood: a systematic review. Int J Obes (Lond) 2011;35:480–492.
37 Satter E: Eating competence: definition and evidence for the Satter Eating Competence Model. J Nutr Educ Behav 2007;39:S142–S153.
38 Dearden KA, Hilton S, Bentley ME, et al: Caregiver verbal encouragement increases food acceptance among Vietnamese toddlers. J Nutr 2009;139:1387–1392.
39 Hurley KM, Cross MB, Hughes SO: A systematic review of responsive feeding and child obesity in high-income countries. J Nutr 2011;141:495–501.

Black RE, Makrides M, Ong KK (eds): Complementary Feeding: Building the Foundations for a Healthy Life. Nestlé Nutr Inst Workshop Ser, vol 87, pp 167–181, (DOI: 10.1159/000449213)

Complementary Feeding in an Obesogenic Environment: Behavioral and Dietary Quality Outcomes and Interventions

Lynne Allison Daniels

School of Exercise and Nutrition Sciences, Faculty of Health, and Institute of Health and Biomedical Innovation, Queensland University of Technology, Kelvin Grove, QLD, Australia

Abstract

The WHO infant feeding guidelines, including those for complementary feeding (CF), are very prescriptive, largely based on the outcomes of exclusive breastfeeding, and have a bias towards undernutrition. Consideration of longer-term outcomes related to overnutrition, the predominant nutrition problem in affluent countries, is limited. Compared to the ongoing and often zealous debates regarding the short- and long-term benefits of exclusive breastfeeding to 6 months in affluent countries, exposures (particularly feeding practices) and outcomes related to CF, independent of exclusive breastfeeding, have received little attention. In this context, consideration of a broader range of outcomes (e.g. food preferences, energy intake regulation, dietary quality, and eating behaviors) that potentially mediate the associations between infant feeding and long-term obesity and chronic disease outcomes is required. The aim of this paper is to (i) consider the impact of CF on outcomes relevant to the risk of child obesity and (ii) provide an overview of the NOURISH trial, the first large trial to evaluate an intervention that specifically targeted CF feeding practices ('how'), including reports on long-term outcomes.

Introduction

The WHO infant feeding guidelines are extremely prescriptive regarding the duration of exclusive breastfeeding and hence introduction of complementary feeding (CF) *'at 6 months of age (180 days)'* [1, p. 10]. These guidelines are predominantly founded on evidence for relatively short-term biological outcomes of exclusive breastfeeding such as growth velocity, infection, and micronutrient status. The emphasis on adequate energy, protein, and micronutrient intake, microbiological safety, active feeding, and frequent meals suggests a bias towards risks of undernutrition [2]. In affluent countries, where the predominant nutrition problem is overnutrition, outcomes related to obesity and chronic disease risk are a priority. Notwithstanding the 'one-size-fits-all' position of the WHO guidelines, consideration of obesity risk outcomes beyond infancy has been limited [2].

Exclusive breastfeeding to and commencement of CF at 6 months are inextricably linked because failing to meet the latter prevents adherence to the former [2]. Compared to the often zealous debates regarding the short- and long-term benefits of exclusive breast feeding to 6 months in affluent countries, CF feeding practices, particularly the 'how', have received little attention in terms of outcomes relevant to the development of food preferences and eating habits that are potentially protective in the excess food environment of affluent countries.

The aims of this paper are to (i) consider the impact of CF practices on behavioral and dietary quality outcomes relevant to the risk of child obesity with a focus on the early phases of CF often termed 'weaning' and (ii) to provide an overview of the NOURISH trial, one of very few early feeding interventions designed to specifically target the process of CF.

Exposures and Outcomes of Complementary Feeding in an 'Obesogenic' Environment

Introduction of solids is far more than the timely provision of energy and nutrients. It is a key developmental milestone that introduces a completely new dimension to the feeding and parenting dynamic. In 2011, Schwartz et al. [3] identified a number of components of CF – 'when, what, and how'. These exposures include timing (initiation and rate of progression); type of food (nutrients, taste, and texture); process (repeated exposure, variety, and self-feeding), and parent feeding practices [control, (non)responsive feeding, and structure]. To date, the focus has been predominantly on the exposures of timing (when) and nutrients (what) and relatively short-term, all be they important, outcomes – growth rate, infection, micronutrient status, atopy, and infant mortality. However, in the affluent country/obesogenic environment context, it is also important to consider a wider range of CF exposures and their associations with dietary quality and eating behavior outcomes that potentially mediate the associations between infant feeding and life-long eating patterns and obesity and chronic disease risk [4, 5]. These 'intermediate' outcomes not only include rapid growth but also taste preferences, food acceptance, and texture tolerance, which are key determinants of early dietary variety and hence quality [4]. Given the developmental importance of this milestone and the critical links between feeding and parenting, outcomes relevant to overall child development and well-being, such as self-regulation, also merit consideration [6, 7].

Influence of Variety at Weaning on Food Preferences, Acceptance, and Intake: Diet Quality

Infants are born with taste predispositions that include rejection of novel foods (neophobia) and bitter/sour and preference for sweet tastes, which once provided an evolutionary advantage, but are no longer adaptive to our contemporary, plentiful food environment [8]. Although these traits have a heritable component, they are also modifiable by the early feeding experience [8, 9]. Improved acceptance of new foods and intake of healthy foods has been demonstrated when, from the introduction of solids onwards, children experience repeated exposure to a wide variety of foods and textures and limited exposure to noncore (high fat/sugar and low nutrient) foods [3, 4, 9, 10]. It appears that neophobia varies with age and is relatively low from 4 to 10 months [10, 11]. Previously, weaning guidelines advised one new food every few days to ensure tolerance. This approach, particularly in the context of exclusive breast feeding to 6 months, may limit the range of foods to which an infant is exposed and accepts before the age-related increase in neophobia. At 4–6 months, daily neutral exposure to a new vegetable (with/without salt) over 10 days resulted in a 2- to 3-fold higher intake independent of the innate preference for salt, with enhanced acceptance in breastfed infants [12]. A French study (n = 203) [11] with detailed concurrent parent reporting on the timing, type, and acceptance (rated on a 4-point scale) of new foods (a total of 171 foods and 38 new vegetables) introduced from a mean age of 5.5 up to 15 months showed that most food categories were generally well accepted. Acceptance ratings increased linearly to 10 months and then plateaued, and for all categories they were positively associated with the number of new foods offered in the first 2 months of weaning. Only for vegetables was earlier introduction associated with better acceptance ratings.

Several papers have investigated the process of introduction of vegetables. Two very detailed studies by Maier et al. [13, 14] examined the impact of high-variety exposure in 147 infants, aged 5.4 months, who had never had any vegetables. High-variety exposure over 9 days comprised once-daily feeding of 3 different vegetables on daily rotation versus feeding each of the 3 vegetables for 3 consecutive days (low variety) or a single vegetable (no variety). High-variety exposure resulted in better subsequent acceptance (g intake at refusal) of the rotated and 2 novel vegetables as well as 2 novel protein foods (pureed meat and fish). In a follow-up study [13] (n = 49, age 7 months), mothers identified one liked and one disliked vegetable (intake 25% of liked) from those used in the previous study. After alternate exposures over 16 days (i.e. 8 exposures each), intake of disliked vegetables increased fourfold (17 g/exposure in a linear fashion) such that g intake to refusal of both vegetables was equal. At age 16 months, based on maternal report, 36 (73%) children were still eating their disliked vegetable, 5 (10%) disliked or refused to eat it, and 7 (15%) had not been offered it again. In a French study, repeated exposure (n = 10 times) to a novel vegetable at 6.4 months of age has been demonstrated to be more effective than flavor-flavor learning (adding sugar) in increasing liking and acceptance for up to 3 months after exposure. Initial acceptance/intake of the novel vegetable was directly associated with the number of vegetables tried before the exposure [15].

Overall, new food acceptance and hence dietary variety may be optimized by ensuring that during weaning infants are repeatedly exposed to as many food categories as possible before neophobia strengthens with age. Few studies have examined the long-term impact of early exposure strategies and variety. We recently demonstrated that the number of fruits, vegetables, and noncore foods 'tried' by 14 months of age was associated with a greater number of foods both liked and consumed within each of these food categories at 3.7 years of age. The exposure experience during the first months of CF (tried more fruit and vegetables and fewer noncore foods) was also directly associated with improved dietary intake and quality at 3.7 years of age. In addition, children who had tried more vegetables at 14 months were reported as less fussy at 3.7 years. These prospective associations were independent of maternal age and education, duration of breastfeeding (weeks), age at solid introduction, maternal BMI, and maternal reported fussiness at 14 months [9]. These data support the hypothesis that variety in early taste and texture experiences influence later dietary quality [4, 8, 10].

Timing of Texture Exposure and Dietary Quality

Data on the impact of feeding practices such as the timing of solid introduction and texture progression on dietary quality are scarce. Two papers [16, 17] provide maternal-report data from 9,360 infants at 6 and 15 months and 7 years of age. The majority of children commenced solids at 3–4 months, consistent with guidelines at that time (1991/1992), but analyses were not controlled for this potential confounder. Introduction to lumpy foods ≥10 months (18% of cohort) was associated with mothers perceiving their child at 15 months and 7 years of age as more difficult to feed and may also have been related to poorer dietary variety and hence quality. There is some evidence that the introduction of lumps prior to 6 months (11% cohort) was associated with benefits related to intake of some categories of vegetable and fussiness, but there was no adjustment for the age of solid introduction per se. A key unanswered question is whether if CF does not start until 6 months are infants able to progress to sufficiently lumpy texture by 9 months of age to avoid the adverse outcomes that appear to be associated with late (>10 months) texture progression?

Timing of Commencement of Complementary Feeding and Diet Quality

Two studies [11, 18] involving large European cohorts reported that age at the introduction of solids had little effect on acceptance/intakes of fruit and vegetables up to 4 years of age. In contrast, in a large, good-quality US study [19], 1,782 mothers (35% eligible) reported every 4–6 weeks (until infant age 12 months) how often their infant consumed 18 food/drink categories over 7 days. Age of solid introduction (<4 months in 41% of infants) was independently associated with increased dietary variety (at least 3 core food groups fed daily over 7 days) at 9–10 months (OR 2.0) and reduced the frequency of intake of high-fat and/or sugar foods at 1 year of age (OR 0.5). These effects were independent of maternal age, education, social disadvantage, race, and breastfeeding at 24–28 weeks. Overall, the albeit very limited evidence suggests that early solid introduction is not associated with poorer dietary quality and may even be associated with improved dietary variety at 12 months.

Multicomponent Interventions

Many correlational studies have suggested that infant feeding practices 'program' taste preferences, texture tolerance, and appetite regulation at a time when both behavior and biology are plastic. In a descriptive study [20] including 361 mothers of healthy children 12–36 months of age, we demonstrated a high prevalence of poor dietary quality and adverse early feeding practices. These included nonresponsive feeding practices that override infant capacity to self-regulate intake and are characterized by excess maternal control through pressure, restriction, or reward and emotional feeding (to calm, distract, and comfort). These practices teach the child to eat for reasons unrelated to appetite. In addition, we confirmed that dietary quality issues were prevalent even in very young children. The seminal 2008 Ventura and Birch [21] review that examined the

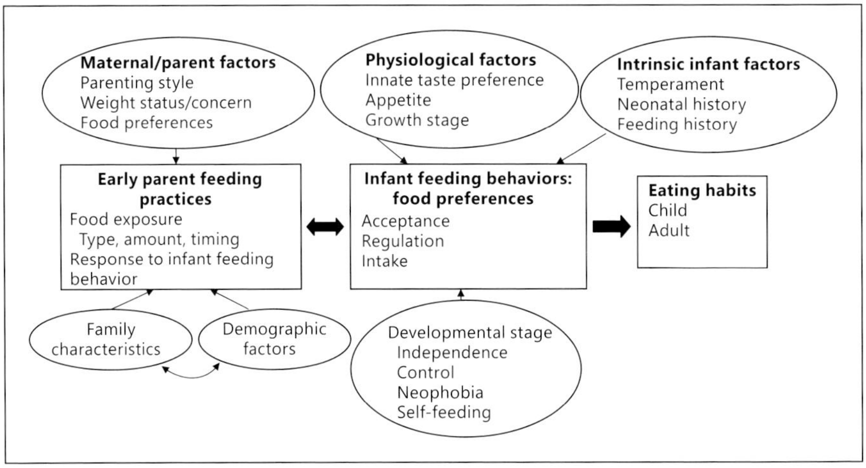

Fig. 1. NOURISH intervention conceptual framework: key factors that influence the reciprocal relationships between parent feeding practices and infant feeding behavior. Neophobia = Rejection of novel foods. Reproduced from Daniels et al. [22] with permission.

role of parenting and feeding practices in child eating behavior and weight status reported only 6/67 studies were longitudinal, none of which included children <5 years old. At that time, there were only two small interventions and neither commenced in infancy [21]. The NOURISH intervention and trial were designed around this time to address this gap [22].

The NOURISH trial [22–24] evaluated a CF intervention for first-time mothers commencing at infant age 3–6 months. The overall research question was *Can anticipatory guidance increase 'protective' feeding practices that support development of healthy child eating behaviors, food intake, and growth?* The overall conceptual framework of the study is shown in figure 1. The protocol, intervention, and outcomes have been reported previously [22–24]. Our clinical experience indicated that once adverse feeding dynamics are established, they are very difficult to change, particularly in the context of autonomy milestones that characterize toddlerhood. As a result, we commenced the intervention at around 4 months of age to enable anticipatory guidance from the start of CF on 'normal' child eating behaviors and positive or protective feeding responses, rather than seeking to manage established problems.

A consecutive sample of first-time mothers of healthy term infants were first approached on postnatal wards. Subsequently, 698 mothers (44% of those recontacted) underwent baseline assessment (infants 4.3 months old) followed by independent concealed randomization. The intervention comprised 2 modules, each of 6 group sessions of 1.5-hour duration delivered over 12 weeks at local child health clinics by study dietitians and psychologists. Module 1 commenced immediately after baseline assessment (children 4.3 months old) and module 2 started 6 months after completion of module 1 (9 months from baseline, children 14 months old). Intervention principles and messages to parents emphasized healthy growth and eating behaviors rather than obesity prevention (summarized in table 1). Table 2 summarizes module session content.

Outcome measures were assessed at 5 time points (table 3). Researchers measured maternal and child weight and length/height at the child health clinics or home visits. Child outcomes included intake (24-hour recall), food preferences, and eating behaviors measured using validated maternal report tools and BMI z-score. Maternal outcomes included feeding practices, strategies to manage food refusal, and parenting skills measured using standard questionnaires. A comprehensive range of covariates included detailed infant feeding data (duration of breastfeeding and age at the introduction of solids), temperament, birth weight (from hospital records), and maternal BMI, education, food preferences, and standard demographics (fig. 1).

The characteristics of the participants have been described in detail elsewhere [24]. Mothers were 30 years old at delivery, 95% were partnered, 58% had a university education, and 78% were born in Australia; 4 months postpartum, BMI was 26. At baseline, infants (51% female) were 4.3 months old, and 57% were fully breastfed, 27% fully formula fed, 34% had been given solids, and mean BMI z-score was –0.31. Average age at solid introduction was 23 weeks. Although there was the expected selection and retention bias according to age, education, partner status, and smoking during pregnancy, there were no differences at baseline or 5 years (T5) according to allocation.

Linear mixed models examined longitudinal group, time, and interaction effects 14 months (T2) to 5 years (T5; table 3), adjusting for baseline values [24]. There was no significant intervention effect on BMI z-score ($p = 0.06$; fig. 2) or prevalence of overweight obesity at T5 (control 13.3% vs. intervention 11.4%; $p = 0.66$). There were significant and sustained intervention effects on self-reported maternal feeding practices from T2 to T5. Intervention mothers used less nonresponsive feeding practices on 6/9 scales ($p < 0.02$). At T5, control mothers were 1.2–1.8 times ($p < 0.05$) more likely to use 7/12 inappropriate (specified) strategies in response to food refusal. Although the intervention effects were maintained to T5, the use of nonprotective feeding practices and counterproductive responses to food refusal increased with child age in both groups. Despite the positive intervention effects on BMI and feeding practices, there were few positive effects on dietary intake/quality or child eating behavior [23]. There were no differences by group in intake of fruits or vegetables (g/kg body weight/day) nor discretionary foods or nonmilk sweetened beverages (% total energy).

Table 1. NOURISH intervention strategies, themes, and parent messages [22]

Evidence-based strategies	Intervention principles	Parent concepts and strategies
Exposure		
Promoting repeated neutral exposure to healthy foods Limiting exposure to unhealthy energy-dense nutrient-poor foods to support development of healthy food preferences [10]	The way we feed young children affects the food they will like and their health Habits are formed early and track to adulthood *Learning to like, liking to eat* [10]	Understand, expect neophobia and innate preferences (salt and sweet) Repeated neutral exposure to healthy foods Limit exposure to sweet, salty foods – covert restriction, role modelling
Responsive feeding		
Recognizing and responding appropriately to child cues of hunger and satiety to support and maintain the child's innate capacity to self-regulate energy intake and avoid overfeeding [33]	Listen to and trust your child *Parents provide, children decide* [33]	Accept food refusal = not hungry or satiety Guide portion size but do not focus on amounts Encourage autonomy – self-feeding to developmental stage and accept mess Neutral response to intake and refusal No coercion, praise, coaxing, and games No rewards, bribes, and alternatives No emotional feeding to distract, comfort, and shape behavior No TV
Positive parenting (warmth, encourage autonomy, and self-efficacy)		
Operationalized via authoritative feeding Characterized by behavioral limits (structure) and maternal sensitivity to cues Decreased overcontrol and -protection [21, 34]	Your relationship with your child is important *Feeding is parenting* Set good examples for your child *Be a good role model*	Provide structure choice – food offered, meal timing and setting (i.e. limits) Provide warmth, encourage independence – responsive to cues and skills Overpowering (authoritarian) – avoid pressure to clean plate Avoid overworrying (permissive or authoritarian) – pressure to eat and overt restriction Don't be a big softie (permissive or unengaged) – as long as they eat something Do not offer alternative or be a short-order cook Feeding is a conversation Allow the child to lead, wait until paying attention; pause for socializing Allow self-feeding and touching food Avoid disruptions – e.g. cleaning face Stop feeding when child loses interest Talk quietly – about the food, encourage but do not coerce, language for hunger/fullness

Table 2. NOURISH intervention module session[a] content

	Module 1 Session	Introducing solids: commenced in children aged 4–7 months *Exposure: Learning to like, liking to eat* [10]
1	Program introduction	Food preferences – innate likes and dislikes, neophobia, Feeding practices – neutral exposure to a wide variety of healthy foods; limit exposure to unhealthy foods Parenting styles and feeding practices Hunger and fullness cues
2	Parenting styles and feeding practices	Parenting styles and attachment, relationship to feeding Feeding practices to support 'attached' feeding
3	Healthy growth and feeding babies	Guide to healthy weight gain Developmental readiness for solids Process for introducing solids Foods to avoid and how much
4	The feeding relationship	'Normal' infant feeding behavior – variable intake and preference for sweet and salty food (limit these); support to try new things, and learn to like new tastes The feeding relationship – conversation, let the child lead
5	Healthy and safe feeding skills	'Listen' to your child, recognize and respond to hunger/satiety cues, offer new foods; limit unhealthy foods Rewards of attached feeding – increases child's confidence and emotional grounding Safe food, use of expressed breast milk and handling and preparation of infant formula
6	Planning for the future	Food refusal is 'normal' – signals satiety – tips to manage; develop language to talk about hunger/fullness Introduction to 'division responsibility' Setting limits and allowing choice within limits
	Module 2 Session	Transition to family food, self-feeding: commenced in children aged 13–16 months Division responsibility: *Parents provide, children decide* [33]
1	Introduction	Toddles are different to babies – they want to be independent; increased neophobia Toddlers do not grow as quickly as babies, they need to eat less Small and highly variable appetites – trust your child to know how much they need to eat
2	Healthy eating	Food groups – number and serve sizes, sample menus: do not focus on amounts Limit 'extra' foods; avoid choking risks Mealtime structure and strategies No TV
3	Parenting styles and feeding practices	Warmth – praise for trying new foods, not for eating Independence – let the child decide how much to eat, self-feeding Overpowering – force-feeding; overworrying – clean the plate 'Big softie' – as long as they eat something

Table 2. Continued

	Module 2 Session	Transition to family food, self-feeding: commenced in children aged 13–16 months Division responsibility: *Parents provide, children decide* [33]
4	Feeding toddlers, understanding autonomy	Adult meals/foods, plan snacks Provide choice within limits – parent decides 'what and when' Treat dessert as part of a meal, manage treats – 'sometimes foods' – when, how often and portion sizes Self-feeding and feeding competence
5	Managing food refusal and fads	Food refusal is normal – satiety, autonomy Regular meals/snacks Realistic amounts, do not offer preferred alternative, especially milk Avoid coercive feeding and excess control Do not use food to shape behavior and avoid emotional feeding (calm, distract, and comfort)
6	Overview, planning for the future	Division responsibility, authoritative feeding and parenting Food away from home/at child care

[a] Modules comprised fortnightly interactive group sessions (n = 10–15/group, duration 1.5 h) facilitated by a dietitian and a psychologist who utilized standardized training and materials developed for the study.

Table 3. Outcome assessment time points, child age, and retention (mothers providing any data) for the NOURISH trial

Outcome assessment	Child age	Time from baseline	Retention[d], (n = 698)
Time 1 (T1)	4 months	Baseline	44%[e]
Time 2 (T2)	14 months	9 months[a]	86%
Time 3 (T3)	24 months	20 months[b]	78%
Time 4 (T4)	45 months	40 months[c]	72%
Time 5 (T5)	60 months	54 months	61%[f]

[a] 6 months after completion of module 1. [b] 6 months after completion of module 2. [c] 2 and 3.5 years after intervention completion. [d] Provided any outcome data. [e] 44% of those able to be recontacted and still eligible. [f] Control n = 211, intervention n = 213.

However, the intervention group showed a higher preference for fruits (75 vs. 69% liked of 16–17 fruits listed; $p < 0.001$) and a healthier fruit and vegetable intake pattern ($p = 0.03$; based on variety and frequency of intake over 24 h and 7 days). There were small significant intervention effects ($p = 0.04$) in the hypothesized directions on the food responsiveness (lower) and satiety responsive-

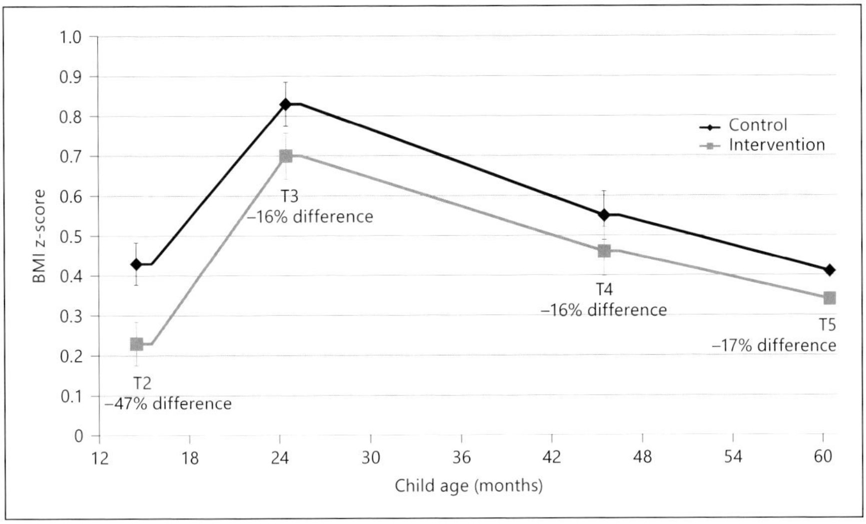

Fig. 2. Longitudinal BMI outcomes (n = 587) of the NOURISH RCT of children aged 14 (T2), 24 (T3), 45 (T4) and 60 months (T5), adjusted for baseline BMI z-score at 4.3 months of age (T1). Linear mixed model (n = 587) using autoregressive structure includes data collected at T2–T5 and adjusted for child BMI z-score at baseline (T1): group effect $p = 0.060$; time $p < 0.001$; group × time $p = 0.57$. Estimated marginal means ± SE. Reproduced from Daniels et al. [24] with permission.

ness (higher) scales from the Child Eating Behaviour Questionnaire, traits that have been positively and negatively associated with weight, respectively [25].

Overall, the results of the NOURISH trial suggest that anticipatory guidance on the process of CF is effective in promoting protective maternal feeding practices and was associated with trends in obesity risk reduction more than 3 years after intervention completion. The impact on dietary quality, food preferences, and child eating behavior was limited.

NOURISH is one of only a few large CONSORT standard trials to evaluate an intervention that specifically targeted feeding practices ('how') related to CF and the first to report long-term outcomes. Although intervention effects on self-reported feeding practices were small, these were seen on most scales used, they were consistent over three time points, and were sustained more than 3.5 years after the end of the intervention. Despite these improved feeding practices, there were no statistically significant effects on anthropometric outcomes. However, intervention BMI z-score was at least 16–17% lower at all four follow-up time points (controlled for baseline), with the overall group effect approaching significance ($p = 0.06$). The two percentage point difference in prevalence of overweight was not significant but at a population level would represent a meaningful public health effect. NOURISH was a universal intervention with participants enrolled regardless of obesity risk. However, exposure to established obesity risk factors such as parental obesity, excess gestational weight gain, formula feeding, and rapid early weight gain may induce epigenetic effects that increase susceptibility to the obesogenic environment [24]. Emerging evidence suggests that heritable traits such as appetite and temperament may influence weight status. Targeting infants with genetic or phenotypic risk may enhance the impact of anticipatory guidance during CF [24, 26]. The attendance at module 2 was disappointing (45% ≥2 sessions), may have dampened intervention response, and suggests the need to consider different formats/approaches to reach mothers of toddlers. The concerning increase in nonresponsive feeding practices in both intervention and control groups across the preschool years suggests parent guidance and support may be beneficial beyond the toddler years [24].

The Early Prevention of Obesity in Childhood: Prospective Meta-Analysis

EPOCH (Early Prevention of Obesity in Childhood) examines pooled individual participant outcome data at 2 years of age from four early feeding trials (from Australia and New Zealand), including NOURISH [27]. The other trials were (i) the Healthy Beginnings Trial (HBT; n = 667) [28], which comprised one prenatal and then six home visits from child health nurses over the first 2 years of life; (ii) the Infant Feeding Activity and Nutrition Trial (InFANT; n = 542) [29], a cluster-randomized controlled trial (RCT) which evaluated six sessions delivered to preexisting groups of mothers with infants 3–18 months old and (iii) PoiNZ [30] (n = 379) which, in addition to seven usual care home visits by child health nurses, delivered eight group sessions, three of which focused on feeding over the first 2 years of life. All trials included first-time mothers only. Analysis (n = 2,196) showed a significant intervention effect on the BMI z-score (–0.12, $p = 0.017$, adjusted for baseline) [31] Like NOURISH [23], InFANT [29] and HBT [28] have reported only limited positive intervention effects on dietary quality with significant differences in the consumption of sweetened beverages (OR 0.48) and snacks (16 g/day) [29], and the prevalence of ≥1 serve of vegetables (89 vs. 83%) [28], respectively. NOURISH is the only trial where the primary intervention focus has been the 'how' of CF and that has reported long-term detailed feeding practice outcomes.

Baby-Led Weaning

Baby-led weaning [32] is an approach to CF that arose from a master's thesis published in 2008 in the lay but not peer-reviewed literature, and is now the subject of numerous online blogs and forums. This approach argues that with the new guidelines to delay solid introduction to 6 months of age, infants are developmentally ready to begin solids by self-feeding 'graspable' family food, and hence spoon-feeding and feeding of purees are not needed at all. However, there is very little research examining the outcome of this approach, and the largely cross-sectional studies that exist are plagued by methodological issues, including defining the extent of baby-led weaning (no versus some spoon-feeding) based on parent report, largely online recruitment, the substantial sociodemographic and breastfeeding practice differences between mothers who do and do not embrace this approach, and the potential for confounding, particularly with exclusive breastfeeding and reverse causality. A large randomized trial (Baby-Led Introduction to SolidS – BLISS) [32] is underway to examine weight status, diet quality, iron and zinc status, energy self-regulation, motor skills, parent feeding practices, acceptability, and adverse outcomes (choking and growth faltering), with outcome assessments at 7,12, and 24 months. Self-feeding supports development of feeding competence and autonomy, and in conjunction with responsive spoon-feeding likely facilitates exposure to a wide variety of foods and textures that supports the transition to a healthy adult eating pattern.

Conclusion

CF is an emotive and contested area of research and practice, at least in part due to the inextricable link with exclusive breast feeding recommendations and the large and persistent gap between policy and practice. It is a key parenting task embedded in culture and tradition, and a source of concern and anxiety for many mothers. There is a clear need for more and better evidence to inform in affluent country guidelines on the 'when, what, and how' of CF based on outcomes relevant to obesity and chronic disease risk. However, there are significant ethical, methodological, feasibility, and funding challenges associated with building this evidence base. The vast majority of mothers do not exclusively breastfeed to 6 months and most mothers commence CF feeding between 4 and 6 months. Mothers need clear and consistent advice on continuing at least some breastfeeding for as long as possible, safe and appropriate bottle-feeding (e.g. avoiding encouragement to empty the bottle), and introducing solids in a way that promotes increased acceptance of a wide range of foods and textures (e.g. repeated, varied exposure, and early texture progression), which preserves the capacity to self-regulate intake (responsive feeding) and supports development of feeding competence and autonomy. There is no doubt that in affluent countries breastfeeding initiation and duration need improving, but this should not be at the expense of research and promotion of optimal timing and process of

CF. There needs to be less political correctness related to exclusive breastfeeding and more research and a stronger focus on optimizing the timing and process of CF.

Acknowledgments

The NOURISH investigators, staff, students, and participants are gratefully acknowledged. Nourish was funded in 2008–2014 by two consecutive grants from the Australian National Health Medical Research Council. Additional funding was provided by H.J. Heinz, Meat & Livestock Australia, Department of Health South Australia, Food Standards Australian New Zealand, and Queensland University of Technology.

Disclosure Statement

We have no financial conflicts of interest relevant to this article to disclose.

References

1 World Health Organization, UNICEF: Complementary Feeding: Report of the Global Consultation, and Summary of Guiding Principles for Complementary Feeding of the Breastfed Child. Geneva, WHO, 2003.
2 Daniels L, Mallan KM, Fildes A, et al: The timing of solid introduction in an 'obesogenic' environment: a narrative review of the evidence and methodological issues. Aust NZ J Public Health 2015;39:366–373.
3 Schwartz C, Scholtens P, Lalanne A, et al: Development of healthy eating habits early in life. Review of recent evidence and selected guidelines. Appetite 2011;7:796–807.
4 Birch L: Child feeding practices and the etiology of obesity. Obesity 2006;14:343–344.
5 Leunissen RWJ, Kerkhof GF, Stijnen T, et al: Timing and tempo of first-year rapid growth in relation to cardiovascular and metabolic risk profile in early adulthood. JAMA 2009; 301:2234–2242.
6 Black MM, Aboud FE: Responsive feeding is embedded in a theoretical framework of responsive parenting. J Nutr 2011;141:490–494.
7 DiSantis K, Hodges E, Johnson S, et al: The role of responsive feeding in overweight during infancy and toddlerhood: a systematic review. Int J Obes 2011;35:480–492.
8 Wardle J, Cooke L: Genetic and environmental determinants of children's food preferences. Br J Nutr 2008;99(suppl 1):S15–S21.
9 Mallan KM, Fildes A, Magarey AM, et al: The relationship between number of fruits, vegetables, and noncore foods tried at age 14 months and food preferences, dietary intake patterns, fussy eating behavior, and weight status at age 3.7 years. J Acad Nutr Diet 2015; 116:630–637.
10 Cooke L: The importance of exposure for healthy eating in childhood: a review. J Hum Nutr Diet 2007;20:294–301.
11 Lange C, Visalli M, Jacob S, et al: Maternal feeding practices during the first year and their impact on infants' acceptance of complementary food. Food Qual Prefer 2013;29: 89–98.
12 Sullivan SA, Birch LL: Infant dietary experience and acceptance of solid foods. Pediatrics 1994;93:271–277.
13 Maier A, Chabanet C, Schaal B, et al: Effects of repeated exposure on acceptance of initially disliked vegetables in 7-month old infants. Food Qual Prefer 2007;18:1023–1032.

14 Maier A, Chabanet C, Schaal B, et al: Breastfeeding and experience with variety early in weaning increase infants' acceptance of new foods for up to two months. Clin Nutr 2008; 27:849–857.
15 Remy E, Issanchou S, Chabanet C, et al: Repeated exposure of infants at complementary feeding to a vegetable purée increases acceptance as effectively as flavor-flavor learning and more effectively than flavor-nutrient learning. J Nutr 2013;143:1194–1200.
16 Coulthard H, Harris G, Emmett P: Delayed introduction of lumpy foods to children during the complementary feeding period affects child's food acceptance and feeding at 7 years of age. Matern Child Nutr 2009;5:75–85.
17 Northstone K, Emmett P, Nethersole F: The effect of age of introduction to lumpy solids on foods eaten and reported feeding difficulties at 6 and 15 months. J Hum Nutr Diet 2001;14:43–54.
18 de Lauzon-Guillain B, Jones L, Oliveira A, et al: The influence of early feeding practices on fruit and vegetable intake among preschool children in 4 European birth cohorts. Am J Clin Nutr 2013;98:804–812.
19 Grummer-Strawn LM, Scanlon KS, Fein SB: Infant feeding and feeding transitions during the first year of life. Pediatrics 2008;122:S36–S42.
20 Chan L, Magarey A, Daniels L: Maternal feeding practices and feeding behaviors of Australian children aged 12–36 months. Matern Child Health J 2011;15:1363–1371.
21 Ventura A, Birch L: Does parenting affect children's eating and weight status? Int J Behav Nutr Phys Act 2008;5:15.
22 Daniels LA, Magarey MA, Battistutta D, et al: The NOURISH randomised control trial: positive feeding practices and food preferences in early childhood – a primary prevention program for childhood obesity. BMC Public Health 2009;9:387.
23 Daniels LA, Mallan KM, Battistutta D, et al: Child eating behavior outcomes of an early feeding intervention to reduce risk indicators for child obesity: the NOURISH RCT. Obesity 2014;22:E104–E111.
24 Daniels LA, Mallan KM, Nicholson JM, et al: An early feeding practices intervention for obesity prevention. Pediatrics 2015;136:e40–e49.
25 Webber L, Hill C, Saxton J, et al: Eating behaviour and weight in children. Int J Obes 2008;33:21–28.
26 Lillycrop KA, Burdge GC: Epigenetic changes in early life and future risk of obesity. Inter J Obes 2011;35:2–83.
27 Askie L, Baur L, Campbell K, et al: The Early Prevention of Obesity in CHildren (EPOCH) Collaboration – an individual patient data prospective meta-analysis. BMC Public Health 2010;10:728.
28 Wen LM, Baur LA, Simpson JM, et al: Effectiveness of home based early intervention on children's BMI at age 2: randomised controlled trial. BMJ 2012;344:e3732.
29 Campbell KJ, Lioret S, McNaughton SA, et al: A parent-focused intervention to reduce infant obesity risk behaviors: a randomized trial. Pediatrics 2013;131:652–660.
30 Taylor BJ, Heath A-LM, Galland BC, et al: Prevention of Overweight in Infancy (POI.nz) study: a randomised controlled trial of sleep, food and activity interventions for preventing overweight from birth. BMC Public Health 2011;11:942.
31 Baur L, Askie L, Rissel C, et al: The Early Prevention of Obesity in CHildren (EPOCH) Collaboration – results of an individual participant data prospective meta-analysis. Obesity Facts 2015;8(suppl 1):5.
32 Daniels L, Heath A-LM, Williams SM, et al: Baby-Led Introduction to SolidS (BLISS) study: a randomised controlled trial of a baby-led approach to complementary feeding. BMC Pediatr 2015;15:179.
33 Satter EM: Internal regulation and the evolution of normal growth as the basis for prevention of obesity in children. J Am Diet Assoc 1996;96:860–864.
34 Patrick H, Nicklas TA, Hughes SO, Morales M: The benefits of authoritative feeding style: caregiver feeding styles and children's food consumption patterns. Appetite 2005;44: 243–249.

Black RE, Makrides M, Ong KK (eds): Complementary Feeding: Building the Foundations for a Healthy Life. Nestlé Nutr Inst Workshop Ser, vol 87, pp 183–196, (DOI: 10.1159/000448966)
Nestec Ltd., Vevey/S. Karger AG., Basel, © 2017

Modifiable Risk Factors and Interventions for Childhood Obesity Prevention within the First 1,000 Days

Anne M. Dattilo

Nestlé Nutrition, Vevey, Switzerland

Abstract

Worldwide, the prevalence of childhood obesity has increased, amounting to 42 million overweight or obese children, and there is increasing evidence that the origins are within the first 1,000 days: the period of conception through 2 years. Antecedents of early childhood obesity are multifactorial, and associations of varying strength have been documented for genetic/epigenetic, biologic, dietary, environmental, social, and behavioral influences. Modifiable factors in pregnancy and early infancy associated with childhood obesity include maternal overweight/obesity, maternal smoking, gestational weight gain, infant and young child feeding, caregiver responsive feeding practices, as well as sleep duration, and physical activity. Promising obesity prevention interventions include those beginning during the first 1,000 days, using a multicomponent approach, with roots in nutrition education theories or behavior change communication that can continue over time. However, the limited number of completed interventions to date (within pediatric clinics or in home-based or community settings) may not be scalable to the magnitude needed for sustainable obesity prevention. Scale-up interventions that can be maintained for the durations needed, addressing infant and young child feeding and other modifiable risk factors associated with childhood obesity are needed.

Introduction

The genesis of childhood obesity is, in part, rooted to the environment within the first 1,000 days, in which nutritional, metabolic, and diet-related behavioral 'programming' is established. Although the general concept of nutritional programming, described as how the nutritional and diet-related environment in utero and during early life affects health at birth and risk of later disease (e.g., fetal origins of disease) is not new [1], recent attention has focused on its role in the prevention of childhood overweight and obesity. Some aspects of nutritional programming may result in frank modulation of organ or endocrine structure and function (e.g., metabolic programming) with lifelong irreversible consequences. However, other aspects of nutritional programming may be corrected (e.g., early flavor programming for later acceptance of taste/flavor) with repeated/learned exposure. Moreover, childhood obesity risks previously deemed to be solely genetic may be a combination of both acquired and environmentally induced effects on gene expression, and some of these epigenetic changes may be modifiable or reversible with appropriate interventions [2].

As the prevalence rates of infant and early childhood overweight (>85th centile) and obesity (>95th centile) are increasing within global populations [2], a rationale has been established to investigate associations between modifiable factors and healthy weight trajectories during the first 1,000 days. Modifiable factors that influence healthy growth of infants, defined as dietary, feeding, and care practices that could be addressed and implemented by the infant's parent(s) and caregivers through interventions beginning at birth, have been identified [3]. Given that obesity from birth through 2 years can persist to childhood [4], predisposing a child to an increased risk into adulthood, there is need to develop interventions with likelihood of success in halting the childhood obesity epidemic, giving particular attention to potential early programming aspects that may be preventable.

Modifiable Factors Associated with Childhood Overweight or Obesity

Multiple genetic, economic, and societal factors have been proposed to explain the global prevalence of childhood obesity. However, several modifiable factors have been identified at the individual level, as maternal and caregiver feeding behaviors, that can be potentially adopted or changed. In general, these factors can be categorized as either food- and diet-related behavior, or feeding and associated lifestyle behaviors (table 1) and have been reviewed in detail elsewhere [3, 5, 6].

Although each of the factors identified has been independently shown to correlate with infant or young child weight, body mass index (BMI), or measures of adiposity, there is increasing recognition that clustering of behaviors is highly likely. For example, evidence suggests a positive association of breastfeeding with maternal responsive feeding practices, which in turn, may have a beneficial effect on a child's self-regulation of eating. For example, mothers of infants breastfed for 3 months reported higher levels of responsiveness to infant hunger and satiety cues than those of infants breastfed for a shorter duration [7]. Early maternal

Table 1. Modifiable dietary- and feeding-related behaviors associated with overweight or obesity in children

Modifiable behavior	Direction of association to overweight or obesity in children
Maternal preconception BMI (as proxy for weight at the time of conception)	Higher maternal BMI before pregnancy has been consistently and positively associated with overweight in infancy or childhood
Gestational weight gain	Excess GWG (categorized as high or in excess of Institute of Medicine recommendations) has been consistently and positively associated with birth weight and risk for infant/child overweight
Maternal tobacco use	Prenatal maternal tobacco smoking has been positively associated with an increased risk of adiposity during childhood
Rate of weight gain during infancy and high infant weight	Rate of weight gain during infancy and/or increased weight for length, BMI, or measurements of adiposity during the first 2 years have been positively associated to BMI and/or adiposity during the toddler or preschool years
Breastfeeding	Breastfeeding duration and/or exclusivity has been inversely associated with rate of weight gain or weight measures during infancy, and with weight, adiposity, or risk of overweight and obesity in toddler and preschool-age children
Age at the introduction of complementary foods	Early age of introduction to complementary foods (e.g., <4 months) has been positively associated with rate of weight gain during infancy and increased weight or measures of adiposity in infants, toddlers, and preschool-age children in some, but not all studies
Diet quality and quantity	
Energy and macronutrient intake	Total energy intake has been positively associated with a higher risk or prevalence of overweight in infant, toddler, and preschool-age children High protein intake has been positively associated with weight gain during infancy and childhood
Intake of sweetened beverages	SSB intake (excluding 100% juice) has been positively related to measures of adiposity or overweight in toddler and preschool-age children
Fruit and vegetable consumption	Children with higher consumption of fruits and/or vegetables, or higher availability of such, consume less total energy and have been associated with a more desirable body composition or body weight during preschool years
Responsive feeding practices	
Attention to 'hunger and satiety cues'	Parental inattention to a child's 'hunger or satiety cues' has been positively associated with overfeeding or overweight in infants
Use of 'controlling', 'rewarding', 'indulgent', or 'restrictive' feeding practices	Parental use of 'controlling', 'rewarding', 'indulgent', or 'restrictive" feeding practices has been associated with the child's food intake, weight gain during infancy, and overweight or obesity in preschool-age children; depending on the parental feeding practice and child's age, the direction of the association has not been consistently reported
TV/screen viewing time	Hours of TV/screen time viewing has been positively associated with overweight or obesity in toddler and preschool age children
Physical activity/active play time	Time spent during physical activity or active play has been inversely associated with measures of adiposity or risk of overweight among infant, toddler, and preschool-age children
Sleep duration	Sleep duration has been inversely associated with overweight, obesity, or measures of adiposity in infants, toddlers, and preschool age children

Table 1. Continued

Modifiable behavior	Direction of association to overweight or obesity in children
Shared family meals/ maternal diet	Frequency of a child's participation in shared family meals per week has been inversely associated with overweight, obesity, or increased risk of overweight in preschool-age children Maternal food intake has been positively associated with toddler diet, at meals and snack time

Adapted from: Woo Baidal et al. [6] (2016); Dattilo et al. [3] (2012), and Weng et al. [5] (2012).

feeding approaches may follow through the period of complementary feeding, with greater maternal responsiveness being related to acceptance of novel foods. As such, multiple diet and feeding behaviors may be interrelated. The degree to which these factors may work synergistically has yet to be identified. Modifiable food and dietary factors associated with infant and childhood overweight or obesity are reviewed below, within a life course framework, as prenatal environmental modifiable factors and infant and young child feeding modifiable factors.

Modifiable Factors within the Prenatal Environment

Prenatal exposures related to maternal overnutrition, such as maternal preconception overweight status and excess gestational weight gain, have been consistently identified to associate with higher infant birth weight or childhood overweight [6]. Glucose control for women with maternal diabetes mellitus, often complicated by overweight or obesity, is also potentially modifiable, and most studies have indicated that gestational diabetes is an independent risk factor for infant or childhood overweight [8]. As discussed below, some evidence supports that diet quality during pregnancy may have an independent effect on infant and young child overweight risk, separate to maternal weight.

Maternal Overweight and Weight Gain during Pregnancy

Women who are overweight or obese at the start of pregnancy (often described as a preconception weight) are at increased risk of developing gestational diabetes mellitus (GDM) and are associated with higher rates of cesarean section delivery, each of which has been independently associated with later childhood risk for overweight. Large-for-gestational-age birth weight (also independently associated with later childhood overweight) is one of several risk factors associated with GDM, and in a retrospective chart review of >9,800 pregnant women, overweight women with GDM were 2.8 times as likely (95% CI: 2.1–3.6) and obese women with GDM were 5.5 times as likely (95% CI: 4.3–6.9) to have a large-for-gestational-age infant as normal-weight women without GDM [8].

Even in the absence of GDM, studies have consistently reported a positive association with maternal BMI and infant birth weight or future childhood obesity risk. Part of this effect is mediated by gestational weight gain (GWG), as maternal overweight has been reported to increase the odds of excessive GWG nearly threefold. Meta-analyses on 12 studies of women with excess GWG indicated an increased risk of childhood obesity (RR: 1.40; 95% CI: 1.23–1.59) from 5 to 18 years of age [9]. Moreover, in a recent prospective cohort study of >100,000 mother-child dyads from two provinces in southern China, the risk of overweight at 3–6 years was doubled in children whose mothers were overweight or obese before pregnancy and experienced excess GWG compared to children of women with adequate preconception weight and recommended GWG (OR 2.22; 95% CI: 1.79–2.76) [10]. Early-, mid-, and late-pregnancy rates of GWG have been independently associated with fat mass and percent neonatal body fat [11], which indicates not only that total weight gain but also that the distribution of weight gain throughout pregnancy contributed to measured adiposity variables at birth. In addition, GWG above the recommended levels was associated with a threefold higher risk of the mother becoming overweight after pregnancy, even among women who were underweight or of average weight before pregnancy [12], perpetuating the likelihood of women entering a subsequent pregnancy at a weight higher than recommended. Given the above consistent relationships, interventions addressing maternal energy intake, and/or adjusting activity, appear as compelling intervention opportunities with promise in prevention of both infant and childhood obesity.

Prenatal Diet Quality

In addition to GWG, strong associations between a high-fat diet and maternal obesity, and obesity in offspring, have been repeatedly recognized in multiple animal models. Some human data have suggested that women who were obese before pregnancy had significantly lower dietary quality scores compared to those with underweight and normal BMI before pregnancy [13], and one recent observational study of 1,079 pregnant women provided evidence that poor maternal diet quality, as assessed by 24-hour dietary recall and a Healthy Eating Index Score, increased neonatal adiposity, independent of maternal BMI before pregnancy and total energy intake [14]. Although additional research is needed to identify specific macronutrient ranges associated with most desirable in utero growth, emerging evidence on diet quality, rather than solely caloric intake or weight gain, further implicates maternal diet as an important exposure for fetal adiposity and the risk for childhood obesity.

'Flavor programming' opportunities offered to the fetus after development of taste buds, via amniotic fluid, from the mother's diet during pregnancy may begin to shape infant food preferences. As such, infants of mothers that consumed carrot-flavored water during the latter part of pregnancy showed preference for carrot-flavored cereal when complementary foods were introduced [15]. A limited number of other flavor compounds (e.g., garlic, anise, and vanilla) have similarly tested positive for infant preference when exposed through the diet of pregnant or lactating women. These findings highlight that the prenatal environment can help modulate not only nutritional and metabolic programming, but via repeated exposure to flavor compounds in utero, infant food preferences may begin to be established.

Modifiable Factors within Infant and Young Child Feeding

The infant diet, beginning with breastfeeding as soon as possible after birth, and timely introduction of nutritious and developmentally appropriate complementary food has long been recognized as a top priority of infant and young child feeding for healthy growth. With regard to childhood obesity prevention, multiple factors related to these concepts are interrelated, including parental responsive feeding approaches, as well as infant behaviors of sleep duration, or sedentary time. The extent to which these associations are independent of each other or due to confounding is unclear.

Breastfeeding

Breastfed infants have shown a different growth trajectory, with typically lower weight gain and less percent body fat than their traditionally formula-fed counterparts [16]. As weight gain during the first year of life is one of the best predictors of later obesity risk [17], a breastfeeding advantage may have long-lasting effects with regard to obesity prevention. Meta-analyses and reviews have concluded that children who had ever been breastfed showed an average risk reduction by 25% for later overweight or obesity. Others have reported that each additional month of breastfeeding resulted in a 4% lower obesity prevalence at later ages.

Many factors, including infant self-regulation of energy intake, caregiver responsive feeding approach, evening feedings, and timing of complementary feeding have been reported to differ between some populations of breastfed and formula-fed infants that might be related to programming of long-term obesity risk. Infants provided formulas with a protein composition similar to breast milk may realize obesity-preventative benefits compared to infants fed formulas with higher protein content [18, 19].

Timing of the Introduction of Complementary Feeding

Multiple systematic reviews, and large observational trials, have not found convincing evidence that introduction of complementary foods between 4 and 6 months of age is associated with an increased risk of overweight or obesity in later infancy, or during early childhood, compared to the introduction of infant feeding at 6 months of age [20, 21]. Results have not been consistent when complementary foods are introduced prior to 4 months.

One systematic review of 23 studies concluded that some evidence suggests that very early introduction (at or before 4 months), rather than at 4–6 months or >6 months, may increase the risk of childhood overweight [21]. However, more recently a nationally representative US study did not support an association between introduction of complementary food intake among infants <4 months of age and parent-reported weight when children reached school age [22], yet a separate large sample from the US with measured weight and length of infants followed up at 2 and 4 years did find a significant effect of timing of complementary feeding on children's weight [23]. Among the latter trial, delaying introduction of solid foods until 4–5 months was associated with lower adjusted obesity odds across 2-year-old children (n = 7,200) and children at 4 years of age (n = 6,950) (OR = 0.67, CI: 0.50–0.89, and OR = 0.66; CI: 0.45–0.98), respectively. Obesity odds were further reduced when complementary food intake delay until 4–5 months was combined with breastfeeding (OR = 0.38, CI: 0.29–0.51, and OR = 0.45; CI: 0.33–0.61 at 2 and 4 years, respectively) [23].

Despite the controversy surrounding the obesity risk if infants are offered solid foods at <4 months of age, few infants will possess the developmentally necessary skills of head, neck, and truncal control to sit with support, and/or have the necessary tongue and swallowing skills to safely manage complementary foods at ages <4 months. Equally important, few infants less than 4 months will likely have the ability to communicate fullness signals to caregivers, compromising their ability to adequately communicate their internal indices of satiation, and increasing the risk of parental overfeeding. As parents often offer complementary foods prior to recommended timing based on their perception that infants are 'old enough', 'baby seemed hungry', or 'it would help baby sleep longer at night', education within interventions addressing these feeding barriers and misconceptions could have meaningful impact on prolonging duration of breastfeeding, and potential prevention of excess energy intake and rate of weight gain among young infants.

Diet Quantity and Quality of Complementary Feeding

Although energy intake has been associated with higher BMI during childhood, limited data are available that specifically assess the effect of energy intake from complementary feeding on subsequent overweight status in children [20, 21]. Within a classic, yet small study [24], energy intake and expenditure were evaluated in 78 primarily formula-fed infants to assess the effect of risk factors at 3 months on overweight/obesity at 1 year. Three-day weighted dietary intake records indicated that energy intake explained a relatively minor (8.0%), yet statistically significant ($p = 0.0002$), influence on weight at 12 months.

Within a larger UK trial [25] that followed 881 infants, energy intake at 4 months was higher in infants who were provided solid foods, and this higher energy intake predicted greater weight gain between birth to 1, 2, or 3 years of age, as well as BMI at 1–5 years. Among formula- or mixed-fed (but not breast-fed) infants, each 420 kJ/day increase in energy at 4 months was associated with an increased odds for being overweight at 3 years (OR: 1.46; 95% CI = 1.20–1.78) and 5 years of age (OR: 1.25, 95% CI = 1.00–1.55).

Results of the US Feeding Infants and Toddlers Study (FITS) in infants from birth to 24 months of age (n = 1,812) [26] consistently showed that infants consumed greater energy intakes throughout the complementary feeding period than the average estimated energy requirement (EER). Measured body weights and heights on the day of the dietary assessment were not available. However, taking median heights and weights for US children as the average weights and heights of the FITS sample, and calculating these EERs, the reported mean energy intakes would exceed the EER by ~8.0–28.0%, depending upon infant or toddler age.

Macronutrient Distribution

Dietary protein intake during infancy, primarily from traditional infant formulas during the first 12 months, has been positively associated with an increased obesity risk and increased BMI during infancy and at 2 and 6 years of age [18, 19]. Infants of overweight mothers may realize particular preventative effects of an infant formula with lower protein content on rate of weight gain, as shown in one randomized controlled trial in which infants provided the experimental formula (1.65 g protein/100 kcal, with probiotics), compared to control formula (2.7 g protein/100 kcal) had slower weight gain between 3 and 6 months, and a significantly lower weight until 2 years [27]. The effect was most striking in infants of obese mothers and in infants with weights >75th percentile, who were already presumed to be at high risk of later obesity. These results add further support to the 'early protein hypothesis', which describes that high protein intake in early life increases plasma and tissue concentrations of insulin-releasing amino acids and stimulates the secretion of insulin and insulin-like growth factor-1 (IGF-1), with resultant increased weight gain and body fat deposition [18].

In a recent review of energy and nutrient intakes of children aged 12–36 months from high-, middle-, and low-income countries around the world, protein intake exceeded the World Health Organization (WHO) reference values in 16 of 17 studies analyzed [28]. Within a further systematic review assessing results from 16 studies with BMI or growth outcome and dietary protein intake data in young children, the authors suggested a mean intake of 15% of energy from total protein as an upper limit for recommended intake at 12 months, as a higher intake may contribute to an increased risk for later obesity [29]. Additional research is needed to establish whether the source of protein (animal, dairy, or total protein) influences obesity risk during infancy and young child populations.

Although the majority of studies have not identified fat intake during infancy or complementary feeding as an independent risk factor for overweight and obesity in later childhood, and one study recognized that in up to 23% of young children's diets the macronutrient distribution range for total fat intake is less than desirable [26], a large prospective cohort study in southeast China reported that fat intake (as fish liver oil) was associated with a greater risk of childhood overweight [30]. Specifically, among 40,510 children in whom anthropometrics were available during infancy and at the 4- to 5-year follow-ups, the early provision of fish liver oil was the only complementary food (of 10 categories) positively associated with follow-up BMI z-scores.

Total carbohydrate intake (from food) during the complementary feeding period has not been positively associated with later adiposity. However, sugar-sweetened beverage (SSB) intake, as a component of carbohydrate intake, has been positively associated with measures of adiposity or overweight in toddlers and preschool-age children, and meta-analyses have established effect sizes ranging from 0.03 to 0.08 unit changes in BMI per 12 fl oz of soda per day, depending upon the length of the follow-up, which varied among studies [3]. One recent study that investigated dietary intake during infancy, and parent-reported weight, identified the prevalence of obesity at 6 years of age among children who consumed SSB during infancy (10–12 months) was twice as high as among non-SSB consumers (17.0 vs. 8.6%, respectively). The adjusted odds of obesity for children who consumed SSB ≥3 times per week were twice that of children who drank no SSB [31].

Within a review of SSB intake in young children, several factors correlated with higher SSB consumption [32], and some could be considered modifiable (e.g., TV viewing/screen time and snack consumption, formula milk feeding, early introduction of solids, parental use of food as rewards, and parental-perceived barriers). Positive parental modeling regarding SSB consumption was consistently associated with lower SSB consumption, suggesting the potential impact of including education around this variable within obesity prevention interventions.

Interventions during the First 1,000 Days Addressing Modifiable Factors for Obesity Prevention

The WHO [2] has recommended that a multifaceted approach be taken to address the current obesogenic environment within low-, middle-, and high-income countries, and that interventions in early life, when biology is most 'plastic' and amenable to change, are likely to have the greatest positive sustained effects on obesity prevention. Regarding behavior changes or the adoption of new behaviors, interventions based on nutrition education theories or behavior change communications hold promise for effectiveness [33, 34]. To date, results from few published multicomponent interventions beginning within the first 1,000 days have reported significant changes in body weight, or measures of adiposity, within a nutrition education randomized controlled clinical trial design.

Utilizing a strict systematic review approach that included interventions implemented during pregnancy or through 24 months of age, with a control group and at least one anthropometric measure of childhood overweight or obesity as an outcome between 6 months and 18 years, Blake-Lamb et al. [35] identified 9 studies that were deemed effective in improving childhood weight status. After eliminating studies that included only infant formula modification as an intervention, one study that was not randomized, and adding an additional study published after their literature search, we present a summary of results from 7 unique trials that utilized multicomponent interventions with significant weight, BMI, or adiposity measures (table 2) [36–45].

Outcome data from the individual studies, performed within multiple global regions, ranged in size from 64 to 598 participants per study. Socioeconomic status of the mother-infant dyads varied, although all interventions were performed in countries with higher economic status. Only one study commenced during the prenatal period, which offered one in-home educational session when women were between 30 and 36 weeks of gestation and followed with 7 intervention visits from birth to 24 months [44].

The majority of studies focused their interventions on a limited number of modifiable factors, such as diet and activity, and one study specifically compared a sleep hygiene and/or introduction to complementary food intervention component [42]. Most studies reported incorporating a nutrition education approach, with a theory-based behavior change or behavior communication strategy within their intervention design (data not shown).

Two studies targeted multiple modifiable factors within a multicomponent intervention approach, including both feeding and feeding-associated behaviors, and each realized initial positive outcomes at 13–15 months [36] and 2 years [44]. These weight outcome differences among intervention and control groups were not sustained at longer-term follow-ups, suggesting that additional intervention time points may have been needed [37, 38, 45]. One common feature, across interventions, was that they were delivered in home, clinic, or community settings. The majority of studies reported utilizing health care professionals or trained personnel to provide the intervention program. All of these pioneer intervention studies [36–45] contributed to our knowledge and understanding of suc-

Table 2. Randomized controlled trials with multicomponent interventions addressing modifiable factors for obesity prevention during the first 1,000 days with significant child weight, BMI, or adiposity outcomes

Author (year) and country of intervention	Population description	Intervention description	Weight, BMI, and adiposity outcomes
Daniels et al. [36–38] (2012, 2013, 2015) NOURISH Trial Australia	Baseline: n = 698 13–15 months: n = 598 2 years: n = 541 5 years: n = 424 First-time mothers	Two 12-week modules (one at 4–7 months and one at 13–16 months) with 6 group sessions in each module Multiple modifiable factors included within the intervention	BMI z-score (control vs. intervention) 13–15 months: 0.42 ± 0.85 vs. 0.23 ± 0.93, p = 0.009 2 years: nonsignificant 5 years: 0.41 ± 0.06 vs. 0.34 ± 0.06, p = 0.06
de Vries et al. [39] (2015) The Netherlands	Baseline: n = 161 Follow-up: n = 143 Infants attending well-baby clinics	1 in-home (at 2 weeks) and 4 clinic-based nurse visits (thru 11 months) Followed to 2.5 years Intervention focus on activity Included dietary advice	Control vs. intervention skinfold thickness: 32.4 ± 6.0 vs. 29.6 ± 4.7 mm, p < 0.05 Females, significantly smaller weight, BMI, and waist and hip circumference
Hakanen et al. [40] (2006) STRIP Trial 10-year follow-up results Finland	Baseline: n = 1,062 10 years: n = 585 Infants at well-baby clinics	Clinic-based, individual counseling 2×/year since infancy Initial dietary intervention on reduced saturated fat intake	Females, lower prevalence of overweight at 10 years (10.2 vs. 18.8%, p = 0.0439)
Mustila et al. [41] (2012) Finland	n = 64	Clinic-based, individual counseling on diet and activity of mothers with infants aged 2–10 months Primary outcome: maternal BMI at 10 months Secondary outcome results on infant weight reported here	Intervention effect on infant BMI z-score at 24–48 months Nonsignificant over full trial course Intervention group: slower increase in BMI z-score (–0.034 to –0.002; p = 0.28 vs. control)
Paul et al. [42] (2011) INSIGHT Trial USA	Baseline: n = 160 Follow-up: n = 110 Mostly well-educated women of higher socioeconomic status	2 × 2 trial, interventions: soothe/sleep and introduction of solids 2 in-home nurse visits at 2–3 weeks and between 4 and 6 months Video and instructional handouts on sleep and feeding	At 12 months, those receiving both interventions had significantly (p = 0.0009) lower mean weight-for-length percentiles (33%), soothe/sleep (50%), introduction to solids (56%), controls (50%)
Verbestel et al. [43] (2014) Belgium	Baseline: n = 203 Analyzed: n = 153 Day care centers Socioeconomic status varied	Tailored feedback for parents on child's activity and diet-related behaviors implemented in day care for children aged 9–24 months	Decrease in BMI z-score from baseline to follow-up (p ≤ 0.05): control (0.74–0.30) vs. intervention (1.38–0.33)
Wen et al. [44, 45] (2012, 2015) Healthy Beginnings Trial Australia	Baseline: n = 667 2 years: n = 497 5 years: n = 369 Low-income, first-time mothers	1 home visit at 30–36 weeks of gestation 7 home visits from birth to 24 months Multiple modifiable factors included within the intervention	BMI difference (control – intervention) 2 years: 0.29 (p = 0.04), 95% CI –0.55, –0.02 5 years: nonsignificant

cessful approaches to educating parents and caregivers on modifiable factors associated with prevention of early childhood obesity.

Utilizing a digitally based technological approach, which has shown promise within interventions among pregnant women and demonstrated effect on behavior with millennial-age women related to breastfeeding, diet, activity, lifestyle, diabetes monitoring, and weight control [46] may help increase short and long term reach, and efficacy of future interventions. In total, outcome data for the 7 trials (table 2) included 2,150 infants/children at the first follow-up. A scale-up approach is needed to extend the reach of such programs globally.

At present, at least 46 trials investigating obesity prevention effects during the first 1,000 days are proposed or ongoing [35]. Approximately 40% of these trials are planned within clinic-based settings, and at least 4 published protocols have included Internet, mobile, telephone, text messaging, or apps as intervention components. To reach, at scale, there is need for future research to assess the impact of well-designed digital interventions compared to other delivery formats.

Conclusion

There is mounting evidence that the origin of childhood obesity is during the first 1,000 days, and modifiable dietary and related lifestyle factors associated with infant and childhood obesity have been identified. Interventions commencing during the prenatal period that include theory-based behavior adoption or behavior change approaches to address maternal diet, gestational weight gain, breastfeeding exclusivity, and timely introduction of nutritious complementary foods are dietary-related components that may influence early programming effects on healthy growth. In combination with other known feeding and lifestyle-related risk factors, multicomponent interventions have a strong rationale for childhood obesity prevention success, yet few interventions have published sustainable results to date. To avoid the limitations of interpersonal interventions which affect coverage, dose, and fidelity, innovative digital and mobile technologies may be one way to extend reach and scale-up efforts that show promise on impacting the childhood obesity epidemic.

Disclosure Statement

Anne M. Dattilo is an employee of Nestlé Nutrition.

References

1 Barker DJ: The fetal and infant origins of adult disease. BMJ 1990;301:1111.
2 World Health Organization: Interim Report of the Commission on Ending Childhood Obesity. Geneva, WHO, 2015.
3 Dattilo AM, Birch L, Krebs NF, et al: Need for early interventions in the prevention of pediatric overweight: a review and upcoming directions. J Obes 2012;2012:123023.
4 Moss BG, Yeaton WH: U.S. children's preschool weight status trajectories: patterns from 9-month, 2-year, and 4-year Early Childhood Longitudinal Study-Birth cohort data. Am J Health Promot 2012;26:172–175.
5 Weng SF, Redsell SA, Swift JA, et al: Systematic review and meta-analyses of risk factors for childhood overweight identifiable during infancy. Arch Dis Child 2012;97:1019–1026.
6 Woo Baidal JA, Locks LM, Cheng ER, et al: Risk factors for childhood obesity in the first 1000 days. Am J Prev Med 2016;pii:S0749-3797(15)00752-7.
7 DiSantis KI, Hodges EA, Fisher JO: The association of breastfeeding duration with later maternal feeding styles in infancy and toddlerhood: a cross-sectional analysis. Int J Behav Nutr Phys Act 2013;10:53.
8 Black MH, Sacks DA, Xiang AH, Lawrence JM: The relative contribution of prepregnancy overweight and obesity, gestational weight gain, and IADPSG-defined gestational diabetes mellitus to fetal overgrowth. Diabetes Care 2013;36:56–62.
9 Mamun AA, Mannan M, Doi SA: Gestational weight gain in relation to offspring obesity over the life course: a systematic review and bias-adjusted meta-analysis. Obes Rev 2014;15:338–347.
10 Guo L, Liu J, Ye R, et al: Gestational weight gain and overweight in children aged 3–6 years. J Epidemiol 2015;25:536–543.
11 Starling AP, Brinton JT, Glueck DH, et al: Associations of maternal BMI and gestational weight gain with neonatal adiposity in the Healthy Start Study. Am J Clin Nutr 2015;101:302–309.
12 Gunderson EP: Childbearing and obesity in women: weight before, during, and after pregnancy. Obstet Gynecol Clin North Am 2009;36:317–332.
13 Shin D, Lee KW, Song WO: Pre-pregnancy weight status is associated with diet quality and nutritional biomarkers during pregnancy. Nutrients 2016;8:162.
14 Shapiro AL, Kaar JL, Crume TL, et al: Maternal diet quality in pregnancy and neonatal adiposity: the Healthy Start Study. Int J Obes (Lond) 2016;40:1056–1062.
15 Mennella JA, Jagnow CP, Beauchamp GK: Prenatal and postnatal flavor learning by human infants. Pediatrics 2001;107:E88.
16 Dewey KG: Growth characteristics of breast-fed compared to formula-fed infants. Biol Neonate 1998;74:94–105.
17 Ong KK, Loos RJ: Rapid infancy weight gain and subsequent obesity: systematic reviews and hopeful suggestions. Acta Paediatr 2006;95:904–908.
18 Koletzko B, von Kries R, Closa R, et al: Can infant feeding choices modulate later obesity risk? Am J Clin Nutr 2009;89:1502S–1508S.
19 Weber M, Grote V, Closa-Monasterolo R, et al: Lower protein content in infant formula reduces BMI and obesity risk at school age: follow-up of a randomized trial. Am J Clin Nutr 2014;99:1041–1051.
20 Grote V, Theurich M, Koletzko B: Do complementary feeding practices predict the later risk of obesity? Curr Opin Clin Nutr Metab Care 2012;15:293–297.
21 Pearce J, Taylor MA, Langley-Evans SC: Timing of the introduction of complementary feeding and risk of childhood obesity: a systematic review. Int J Obes (Lond) 2013;37:1295–1306.
22 Barrera CM, Perrine CG, Li R, Scanlon KS: Age at introduction to solid foods and child obesity at 6 years. Child Obes 2016;12:188–192.
23 Moss BG, Yeaton WH: Early childhood healthy and obese weight status: potentially protective benefits of breastfeeding and delaying solid foods. Matern Child Health J 2014;18:1224–1232.
24 Stunkard AJ, Berkowitz RI, Stallings VA, Schoeller DA: Energy intake, not energy output, is a determinant of body size in infants. Am J Clin Nutr 1999;69:524–530.

25 Ong KK, Emmett PM, Noble S, et al: Dietary energy intake at the age of 4 months predicts postnatal weight gain and childhood body mass index. Pediatrics 2006;117:e503–e508.
26 Butte NF, Fox MK, Briefel RR, et al: Nutrient intakes of US infants, toddlers, and preschoolers meet or exceed dietary reference intakes. J Am Diet Assoc 2010;110:S27–S37.
27 Inostroza J, Haschke F, Steenhout P, et al: Low-protein formula slows weight gain in infants of overweight mothers. J Pediatr Gastroenterol Nutr 2014;59:70–77.
28 Suthutvoravut U, Abiodun PO, Chomtho S, et al: Composition of follow-up formula for young children aged 12–36 months: recommendations of an international expert group coordinated by the Nutrition Association of Thailand and the Early Nutrition Academy. Ann Nutr Metab 2015;67:119–132.
29 Hornell A, Lagstrom H, Lande B, Thorsdottir I: Protein intake from 0 to 18 years of age and its relation to health: a systematic literature review for the 5th Nordic Nutrition Recommendations. Food Nutr Res 2013;57:10.3402/fnr.v57i0.21083.
30 Zheng JS, Liu H, Zhao YM, et al: Complementary feeding and childhood adiposity in preschool-aged children in a large Chinese cohort. J Pediatr 2015;166:326–331.
31 Pan L, Li R, Park S, et al: A longitudinal analysis of sugar-sweetened beverage intake in infancy and obesity at 6 years. Pediatrics 2014;134(suppl 1):S29–S35.
32 Mazarello Paes V, Hesketh K, O'Malley C, et al: Determinants of sugar-sweetened beverage consumption in young children: a systematic review. Obes Rev 2015;16:903–913.
33 Contento IR: Nutrition education: linking research, theory, and practice. Asia Pac J Clin Nutr 2008;17(suppl 1):176–179.
34 World Health Organization: Health Education: Theoretical Concepts, Effective Strategies and Core Competencies: A Foundation Document to Guide Capacity Development of Health Educators. Geneva, WHO, 2012.
35 Blake-Lamb TL, Locks LM, Perkins ME, et al: Interventions for childhood obesity in the first 1,000 days: a systematic review. Am J Prev Med 2016;50:780–789.
36 Daniels LA, Mallan KM, Battistutta D, et al: Evaluation of an intervention to promote protective infant feeding practices to prevent childhood obesity: outcomes of the NOURISH RCT at 14 months of age and 6 months post the first of two intervention modules. Int J Obes (Lond) 2012;36:1292–1298.
37 Daniels LA, Mallan KM, Nicholson JM, et al: Outcomes of an early feeding practices intervention to prevent childhood obesity. Pediatrics 2013;132:e109–e118.
38 Daniels LA, Mallan KM, Nicholson JM, et al: An early feeding practices intervention for obesity prevention. Pediatrics 2015;136:e40–e49.
39 de Vries AG, Huiting HG, van den Heuvel ER, et al: An activity stimulation programme during a child's first year reduces some indicators of adiposity at the age of two-and-a-half. Acta Paediatr 2015;104:414–421.
40 Hakanen M, Lagstrom H, Kaitosaari T, et al: Development of overweight in an atherosclerosis prevention trial starting in early childhood. The STRIP study. Int J Obes (Lond) 2006;30:618–626.
41 Mustila T, Raitanen J, Keskinen P, et al: Lifestyle counselling targeting infant's mother during the child's first year and offspring weight development until 4 years of age: a follow-up study of a cluster RCT. BMJ Open 2012;2:e000624.
42 Paul IM, Savage JS, Anzman SL, et al: Preventing obesity during infancy: a pilot study. Obesity (Silver Spring) 2011;19:353–361.
43 Verbestel V, De Coen V, Van Winckel M, et al: Prevention of overweight in children younger than 2 years old: a pilot cluster-randomized controlled trial. Public Health Nutr 2014;17:1384–1392.
44 Wen LM, Baur LA, Simpson JM, et al: Effectiveness of home based early intervention on children's BMI at age 2: randomised controlled trial. BMJ 2012;344:e3732.
45 Wen LM, Baur LA, Simpson JM, et al: Sustainability of effects of an early childhood obesity prevention trial over time: a further 3-year follow-up of the Healthy Beginnings Trial. JAMA Pediatr 2015;169:543–551.
46 Willcox JC, van der Pligt P, Ball K, et al: Views of women and health professionals on mHealth lifestyle interventions in pregnancy: a qualitative investigation. JMIR Mhealth Uhealth 2015;3:e99.

Black RE, Makrides M, Ong KK (eds): Complementary Feeding: Building the Foundations for a Healthy Life. Nestlé Nutr Inst Workshop Ser, vol 87, pp 197–199, (DOI: 10.1159/000448977)

Summary of Factors Influencing Healthy Growth

The third session considered factors around the complementary feeding stage that influence healthy growth and development with an emphasis on the prevention of obesity and the establishment of healthy eating habits. While this has long been considered to be an issue predominantly for western settings, obesity is becoming a global problem that often begins in childhood, and many developing settings pose the challenge of setting food policies that consider the double burden of coprevalent under- and overnutrition. In this context, it was welcome to hear how the same principles of food responsiveness may be applicable to the management of both poor infant feeding and to rapid infant weight gain, too. However, considering the health relevance of the infant growth rate, it is essential to have a clear understanding of the population context in terms of the prevalence of childhood underweight/stunting and overweight.

Ken K. Ong described that mortality from noncommunicable diseases is higher in UK 65-year-olds who had experienced early life growth stunting – this has important implications for long-term health in current childhood populations in whom stunting remains common. Conversely, many contemporary western birth cohorts now show rates of infancy weight gain and energy intakes far above the WHO growth standard, and Ong described the wealth of evidence linking these trajectories to later life obesity. When considering the possible underlying mechanisms, it is important to recognize that infant feeding is the result of a complex interaction and signaling between the mother and infant – hence, both infant and maternal factors need to be understood. There is increasing evidence that common 'genetic variants of obesity susceptibility' affect weight gain during infancy and childhood – the higher attained weight persists through life with adverse consequences for adult obesity, diabetes, and other obesity-related metabolic disorders. Furthermore, these variants appear to act through central mechanisms that influence infant appetitive constructs relating to food (appetite) or satiety responsiveness, which in turn show significant heritability, and are predictive of infant weight gain and later body size.

Maureen M. Black and *Kristen M. Hurley* gave an illuminating analysis of the roles of both child and parent in infant feeding, and the translation of this understanding into strategies to promote healthy mealtime interactions. Responsive feeding is a derivative of responsive parenting and recognizes the reciprocity between the parent and child during feeding. Parents need to recognize feeding cues from the child, and learn to respond in a prompt, emotionally supportive manner – and to find the right balance between demandingness (the parent in charge) and nurturance (the child in charge). Furthermore, both the interactions and the feeding behaviors change rapidly during infancy, and responsive feeding needs to be contingent and developmentally appropriate. They described how interventions based on responsive feeding were widely promoted to manage issues of infant food refusal, food selectivity (pickiness), or disruptive mealtime behavior, and more recently have been used to develop behavioral interventions against overweight.

Lynne A. Daniels described how recent studies have embedded principles of food responsiveness into interventions to prevent rapid infant weight gain and childhood obesity. In contrast to earlier approaches that focused on exposures of timing and type of nutrients with relatively short-term outcomes, she highlighted the importance of going beyond rapid growth, to promote resilience to the obesogenic environment through taste preferences, food acceptance, and texture tolerance, which are key determinants of early dietary variety and diet quality. She described that the NOURISH trial demonstrated that anticipatory guidance on the process of complementary feeding increased protective maternal feeding practices and was associated with near-significant trends in obesity risk reduction >3 years after intervention. While some large US trials are still ongoing, she described highly encouraging findings from EPOCH, the Antipodean collaborative meta-analysis across four infant feeding trials to prevent rapid weight gain and obesity. This is a relatively new field, but with much activity. We look forward to future publications of EPOCH, to the findings of the US trials, and to considerations of whether such interventions should be applied universally or targeted to high-risk groups.

Finally, *Anne M. Dattilo* provided an important perspective on how such focused intervention on infant feeding behaviors might fit within a wider strategy that considers other potential modifiable influences within the first 1,000 days to prevent childhood obesity. There is now consistent evidence from observational studies for both in utero or early postnatal factors, which can be broadly categorized as food- and diet-related behaviors, or feeding and associated lifestyle behaviors. For behavior change, or adoption of new behaviors, interventions based on nutrition education theories or behavior change communications hold promise for effectiveness. These targets are being increasingly tested in multicomponent interventions, and the results of these studies have been reviewed, indicating a number of effective interventions. However, to date, most have targeted individual or family level changes in clinical settings rather than early-life systems and policies – hence it will be important to translate these effective approaches to sustainable and potentially scalable strategies to reach large populations.

Ken K. Ong

Subject Index